Pretend
Your Nose
Is a
Crayon

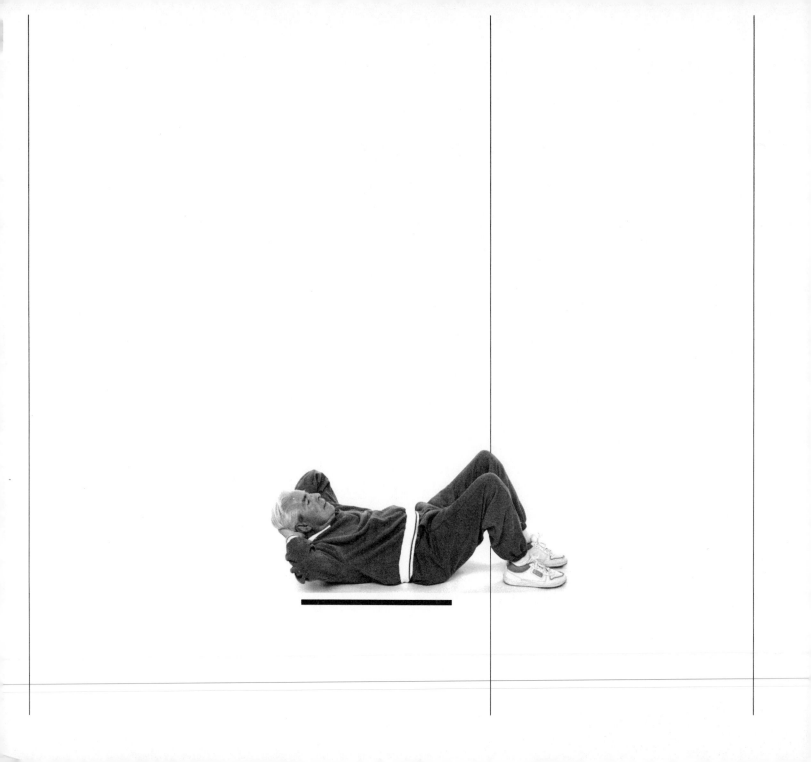

Carol Greenberg with Sara Stein

Pretend Your Nose Is a Crayon

A N D

OTHER STRATEGIES

F O R

STAYING YOUNGER

LONGER

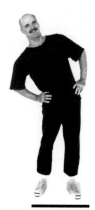

Houghton Mifflin Company
Boston   1991

For information about permission to reproduce selections
from this book, write to Permissions, Houghton Mifflin
Company, 2 Park Street, Boston, Massachusetts 02108.

Library of Congress Cataloging-in-Publication Data
Greenberg, Carol (Carol S.)
   Pretend your nose is a crayon and other strategies for staying
younger longer / Carol Greenberg with Sara Stein.
       p.   cm.
   ISBN 0-395-55741-0. — ISBN 0-395-55742-9 (pbk.)
   1. Physical fitness. 2. Exercise. 3. Physical fitness for the
aged. 4. Exercise for the aged.   I. Stein, Sara Bonnett.
II. Title.
GV481.G73   1991   90-25025
613.7′0449 — dc20   CIP

Printed in the United States of America

CRW 10 9 8 7 6 5 4 3 2 1

Book design by Jennie Bush, Designworks, Inc.

To my fabulous son, Josh,

my mentor, Dorthy Levinson,

and to all of my patients,

who made this book a reality

Contents

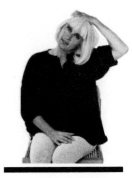

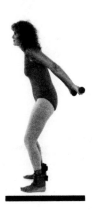

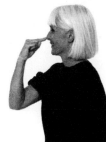

The characters in this book are real — not professional models or fitness experts, but friends, friends of friends, and relatives of mine and Sara's who were kind enough to spend many hours posing for the photographs.

Martin Stein, Sara's husband, is an architect approaching his sixtieth birthday who gardens, clears land, splits wood, and builds stone walls on weekends.

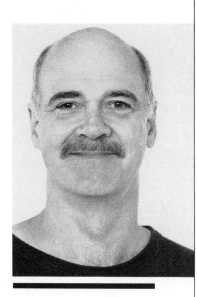

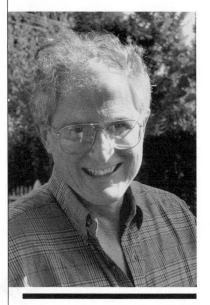

Gloria May is a particularly dear friend. She was a ballet dancer once upon a time and now manages her own gift basket business in Boston. Gloria runs daily and also bikes, camps, and enjoys whitewater rafting and fly-fishing. She has just turned fifty.

Peter Watts is a clinical social worker in his late fifties — and an old friend of mine. Besides canoeing, his favorite activity is repairing and restoring a splendid Victorian home in Connecticut.

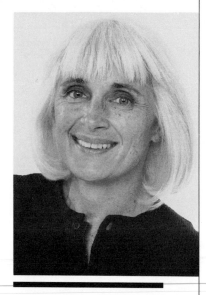

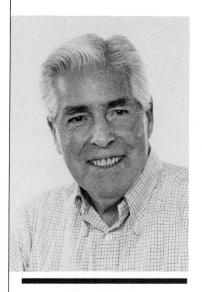

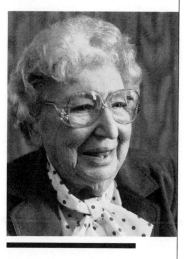

Sara Levenson, Sara's aunt, is ninety-four years old. She has remained active in civic affairs in her home town of Elizabeth, New Jersey, maintains her own apartment, and lives alone.

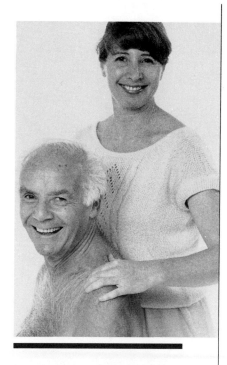

David Smith has been a marketing consultant throughout his professional life and has no intention of retiring. He has won four senior national championships in squash tennis, is currently ranked number two in the East in singles for players over seventy, and is also nationally ranked.

Carol Taylor is a massage therapist, and her partner in the photographs, Herman Mayers, is a retired butcher. Herman, seventy-five, plays paddleball three times a week.

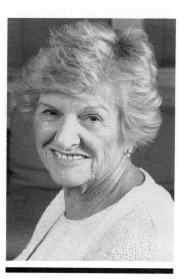

Thelma Parker is my beloved aunt. At seventy-two, she keeps in shape by attending exercise class every morning; she also helps to care for several grandchildren.

All of you, thank you very much for your time, patience, good cheer, and — most of all — for providing photographic evidence that you have stayed younger longer!

Carol Greenberg
October 1990

Pretend
Your Nose
Is a
Crayon

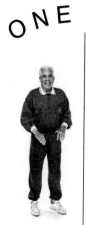

ONE

Darling, We Are Growing Older

T he first lines of the golden oldie from which I paraphrased this opening title are really "Darling, we are growing old, silver hairs among the gold." Well, I'm not about to give up my golden locks, and I'm not ready to grow old.

I will admit to growing older. Who can deny the obvious?

Check it out for yourself. Haven't stairs gotten steeper? Suitcases heavier? Don't you hesitate before sprinting for the bus? Maybe you ache when you wake up in the morning. Maybe your knees object to being kneeled on. Does your wedding ring still slip easily past your knuckle? Can you still show off your biceps the way you used to on the beach?

Or try this test: Pretend your nose is a crayon. Write your name with it. If you hear crackling noises in your neck, that's a sure sign of aging. If you don't, it's only a matter of time.

The Question of Time

The question is how much time: How much time until you have to give up pleasures you now enjoy; how much time until your independence begins to slip away. These days, when we can expect to live longer than previous generations did, the frailty of old age looms large, and almost everybody worries about it sometimes.

This book is designed to ease these worries by showing you how to delay, and even reverse, the effects of aging. You'll still get older, and a day will come when you'll be weaker and creakier than you are, but less so, less fast, than if you did nothing but prepare the rocking chair.

Yes, aging is inevitable. But some people age faster than others, and not only on the outside, but to their very bones. You'll notice that doctors always ask your age. They have to; no examination, blood test, x-ray, or chemical analysis can distinguish between a decrepit sixty-year-old and a spry octogenarian. Until recently, it was thought that differing rates of physical aging were written in the genes. "If you want to live to be a hundred," went the quip, "choose your parents wisely." Doctors are coming to realize — and scores of studies support — that the rate at which people age depends as much on how they lead their lives as on their genes. You *can* slow the clock. You *can* turn it back. And you don't have to pant and sweat to do it.

Staying strong and limber — and altogether healthier by any measurement — doesn't require the physical punishment and fanatic endurance that run the younger crowd to fitness. If you're over fifty, such regimes are more likely to send you to the doctor than to rejuvenation. I have spent twenty-five years as a physical therapist treating the pains and injuries of patients who crazily harbor the ambitions of a twenty-year-old in a body three times that age and, on the other hand, of patients who accept the infirmities of old age in a body barely sixty. The trick to slowing down the aging process without having to emulate Jane Fonda or the late Jim Fixx is to simply not sit still for it.

I'm going to ask you to move — to stretch your joints, flex your muscles, stand tall, and walk. Don't worry that this regime doesn't take your breath away; it's enough to work, not enough to hurt.

Aging can be a downward spiral in which the first cricks and twinges lead people to move less, and so to become stiffer and weaker still. Frailness, in turn, leads people to distrust their sense of balance, to anticipate the stinging pain, the buckling joint, to walk with shorter steps, at a slower pace, to no longer reach so far, or lift so much, or try so hard. The bands that hold flesh and bone together shorten as they become rigid. Muscles lose tensile strength as they lose power. Bones unstressed by muscular effort become porous and brittle. Those who yield entirely invite injury — spasms, tears — when they ask of their fibers feats they no longer have the suppleness or strength to perform. Or they fall and break.

And that's not all. Circulation, respiration, blood pressure, and metabolism are all compromised by inactivity — not to mention that infirmity is downright depressing. Depression is the very pit of the downward spiral, and it looks more and more as if a decline in immunity and memory — the double whammy of getting sick and feeling stupid — are related to how glum a person is.

These changes are insidious at first. The snap, crackle, and pop that eventually will inform you that your joints are aging are caused by a number of subtle changes that, if you're sitting there smugly at thirty, are happening to you already. Nasty little molecules that come to you in foods that are browned or toasted — and even in the normal air you breathe — are glomming onto ligaments and tendons, binding their fibers tight, stiffening them like rubber baking in the sun. Every minute you sit, microscopic telescoping assemblies that contract your muscles are falling apart, leaving you a little weaker than you were. Funny-looking bone-building cells — rotund critters that walk through bones on stumpy stalks — are lazing around, convinced by the lack of pressure on their product that they can take a rest. Fibroblasts, spiky cells that spin your connective tissues, are aging as fast as you are. The salty fluid that plumps their fabric and cushions joints is drying up. Right now, in your shoulders, the glistening white, tough,

What's All the Noise About?

Joints are like any mechanical device. Parts move in relation to other parts, and if they are to move silently, they must fit neatly with one another, and surfaces must be smooth and well oiled to reduce friction. The noisiness of aging joints is the creak of tendons as they slide across rough spots, the crackle of pitted joint surfaces that neither fit so well nor are so lubricated as they used to be. Put your ear to a fifty-year-old knee as it is bent and straightened to hear the noise. Most of the time, a joint's bark is worse than its bite. Knees can creak quite painlessly.

springy surface that lets your arms swing smoothly in their sockets is thinning over the crunchy bone below. Feel it?

Now, bend your arms like chicken wings and slowly flap — up, back, and down again. Hang your arms loose, and shrug your shoulders — up, back, down, and forward in a slow circle, and then again the other way — up, forward, down, and back. Feel better? Your joints are better too.

Such simple stretching exercises, as luxurious and as pleasurable as a yawn, ease stiffening fibers, awaken their makers to their spinning duties, and get joint juices flowing. My easy limbering routine is both a preventive and an antidote to the creaks. And, since most stretches are as unobtrusive as shrugs and yawns, you can do them anytime, anywhere. A stretch takes only seconds.

Stretching specifically lubricates joints and eases the straps and collars that may limit their movements. It hasn't much effect on muscle strength. The cells that form skeletal muscles — the ones that make the skeleton inside you jiggle and dance — can't reproduce. The ones you have now are all you're ever going to have. But they continue through-

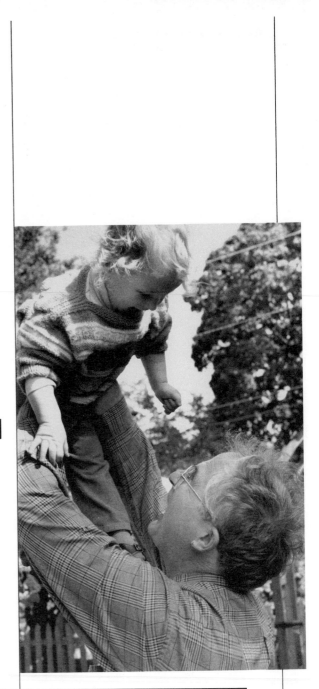

Fitness Four Ways

This four-way fitness program exercises your body in a balanced way. Stretches limber you; isometrics firm your muscles; weight training strengthens you; walking gives you physical endurance. The program is moderate as well as balanced. It avoids activities that could damage joints; it asks only a level of activity that is comfortable for you. You can therefore start this program at any age — grandparent, even great-grandparent — and still enjoy tangible and surprisingly rapid gains in flexibility, firmness, strength, and endurance.

out life to manufacture and discard the telescoping units that contract them and that are, in effect, your strength. Muscles are just dumb meat, as obedient as oxen, but disinclined to work unless prodded into action. You, the brain of this whole operation called your body, are the prodder. If you lie down for a week, you'll weaken, and your muscles will be measurably smaller than they are now. Unworked muscles trash their neglected machinery and don't bother to replace it.

Two kinds of activity prod muscles to manufacture contractile machinery. Isometrics makes them maintain the status quo: They don't get bulgy, but they don't thin to limp spaghetti, either. An isometric exercise uses muscles without moving joints. Put your open palm against your temple, and press head and palm against each other for a couple of seconds. Your arm and neck muscles learn from the pressure the minimum effort you expect of them.

Building muscle is another story. It requires movement and more work than the muscle is accustomed to doing. If a muscle isn't asked to put forth extra effort, it won't build up extra strength. I suggest weights — dumbbells for the hands and sandbags that fit around the ankles — to strengthen limbs and trunk, and a few other exercises to strengthen major muscles.

In addition to stretches, isometrics, and minimal (but sufficient) strengthening exercises, only one other sort of activity is needed to slow the body's aging: walking. Fitness for the young has become synonymous with aerobic fitness — the ability of the circulatory system to deliver oxygen copiously to skeletal muscles as they work, or, in common terms, to be able to climb from the subway without panting. You don't have to run and jump for that. Just a good walk, enough to warm you up and make you breathe more briskly, is enough.

Walking is the dessert on this fitness menu. Too often people walk as though they were wind-up toys geared only to put-put along the pavement. Arms are made to swing, feet to flex, knees to bend, hips to swivel, heads to look at sights more interesting than the sidewalk straight ahead. The stretch and exercise routine will give you the strength and flexibility to stride freely; the chapter on pace and posture will help you *feel* your stride from lifted head through tucked-in gut to springing feet. That's pleasure, not just aerobics. And good posture will help to rid you of the aches.

See Your Doctor First

Fitness books are like cookbooks for some people: They can't wait to try them out. I don't want you to start this fitness regime until you check it out with — and preferably also get a checkup from — your doctor. In New York State, where I practice, patients can't just walk in off the street into my office for a fitness program or for any kind of therapy. First, the person has to be examined by a doctor. Then the patient, accompanied by a prescription for exercise and sometimes an envelope of x-rays, comes to me for treatment. So just because I'm a physical therapist doesn't mean you can trust that every exercise I suggest for people over fifty in general is safe specifically for you. I've never seen your x-rays; your doctor has never told me anything about your heart or blood pressure. I can't even ask you where you hurt.

Hurt is what I see in my profession. Unnecessary hurt. Crazy hurt. Awful damage to bodies in no shape to take the risks and burdens placed on them by their aging owners. I'm going to tell you several cautionary tales in hopes that you might see yourself in one of them and mend your ways.

There's the man who ran the hills of Corfu. He was fat and more than fiftyish, and he limped into my office with a knee the size of a football. What had happened to him? He didn't know and couldn't understand it; he thought he'd get in a little basic training, like back at Fort Dix, where they whipped you into shape in just about the length of time he had for a vacation on Corfu. Never mind that his knee had been complaining for some months about the brief weekend jogs that were his only form of exercise. He really thought that pounding the knee still

Complaint List

Perhaps you've been noticing some small discomfort, such as a knee that sometimes catches, an ache below a shoulder, or a pain when you twist your wrist a certain way. These are the minor complaints that, when one is talking with a busy doctor, can easily slip the mind. However, a minor complaint can be an early warning of worse to come if nothing is done about it. Write down small discomforts as you notice them. Take your complaint list along when you go to see your doctor.

harder was going to get it into shape, but a football wasn't the shape he had in mind.

Human knees and backs are evidence that if there is a Great Maker in the sky, he or she is a lousy engineer. Human anatomy is a makeshift adaptation of what was originally a four-footed design. Putting a quadruped up on two feet doubles the pull of gravity on the legs and spine. When that burden is multiplied by pounding the pavement, knees are going to feel it, and when back muscles aren't strong enough to share the strain, something's got to give. Every joint in the body, no matter how nicely it's been treated, eventually suffers wear and tear that can't be mended. The hills of Corfu are no place for the fat and fiftyish to pursue their youth.

On the other hand, idleness also leads to disability. Witness the little old lady, apparently in her eighties, who hobbled in one day on the arm of her companion. For years she hadn't been able to walk two blocks to a grocery store, to carry a bag of groceries, or to cook a meal. She was depressed and in constant pain; she complained of lack of balance and feared the wind might blow her over. The awful thing is, this "old lady" was only sixty-two.

What ailed her was the creeping weakness of muscles that had never been called upon to do much of anything. Strengthening exercises worked wonders. Now she walks, she carries, she cooks and

A Sexist Observation

Imagine two people, each suffering a backache. One takes to bed, the other to the jogging track. Based on years of observing patients' responses to pain, I'd guess the one lying down is most likely a woman, the one running around is most likely a man. Women tend to protect their body when it hurts; men tend to test it further. My own objective view is that both treatments arise equally from worry: One sex reasons that if the back hurts, it can't be moved; the other reasons that if the back can move, it can't be hurt. Both are wrong. Underuse and overuse are equally risky treatments for joint and muscle injuries, and a doctor's opinion is much more reliable than either sex's inner voice.

cleans, and the companion has long since been dismissed. The last I heard from this little old lady, now in her mid-seventies, was a postcard from Europe, where she was traveling energetically, cheerfully, painlessly, and on her own.

Seventy percent of my patients come in with back pain, mostly brought on by months or years of weakening disuse followed by a spurt of damaging overuse. There was the man who emerged from a winter of passive sport in front of the television to take down the storm windows; he threw his back into spasm, fell off the ladder, and broke his shoulder. That was a clear case of seasonal unfitness. And it doesn't take juggling windows to strain a back softened by a winter on the couch. Another patient, a woman, went into spasm while lifting a can of tomatoes out of a grocery bag. Though most back cases can be cured by exercise to strengthen muscles, it would have been easier to keep the backs strong in the first place.

But not always. This last of my parables is the hardest to grasp because at first it doesn't seem that there's a lesson to be learned.

One day a crisp, straight-haired survivor of the sixties generation hobbled in demanding a cure for her back, which, accustomed to three decades of carrying her photographic gear, had at last rebelled. This aging flower child, wearing a Laura Ashley dress that would have looked cute on her daughter, exemplifies the subtlest kind of craziness that keeps physiotherapists in business. She had been led to believe that if you were a good girl — ate the right food, did the right exercises — you'd stay just that: a girl.

It isn't so. You can't do at seventy what you did at thirty even if you've been the goodest girl in the world.

Aging is real, not to be abused by either the psychic paralysis that turns a sixty-two-year-old woman into an invalid or the insane denial that prompts a couch potato to juggle windows on a ladder. The photographer learned to lighten her gear and take the middle road to fitness. She — and all of us who, in spite of some reluctance to count our silver hairs, are willing to face the facts — can stride into our eighties suitably slowed, but actively independent.

Good Sports

Like doctors, physical therapists have specialties. Mine is sports injuries. So let me advise you about sports.

Whatever you play, don't play so hard. The cost of winning at all costs is awful injuries that amount to self-abuse. Play with friends, not rivals. Play with them, not against them. Play up to the point of tiredness, not beyond. Stop if you hurt.

Whenever you play, warm up first. Cold muscles and stiff joints tear more easily than warmed muscles and stretched joints. Each sport has a warm-up routine that you can learn from books or pros if you don't know it already.

However much you play, exercise too. Most sports, in most parts of the country, are seasonal. Sports injuries peak in winter with ski injuries and again in spring with tennis, golf, and running injuries. By no accident, these peaks come early in their respective seasons, when people are out of shape from the previous season's sloth. Much damage could be avoided by exercising to keep the body fit throughout the year in preparation for the sudden onslaught of the sporting season.

And beware: Running pounds knees. Skiing breaks bones. Tennis twists knees, ankles, elbows, and wrists. Golf strains backs and shoulders and twists elbows too.

Or choose to swim, to row, to paddle a canoe, to dance, to bowl, to play volleyball, badminton, softball, horseshoes, or croquet. I've never seen a croquet injury ever, even though the game is known to be as fiercely competitive as tennis.

Croquet, anyone?

The Hard Facts

In case you're hankering for data about the aging process, here's a smattering of statistics culled from an article by Jane E. Brody for the *New York Times*.

Physiological maturity is reached by about the age of twenty-five. Physiological decline begins by the age of thirty. From then on, the heart's pumping ability declines by 1 percent a year. Blood vessels are nearly 30 percent narrower by middle age. By sixty, blood flow from the limbs is 30 to 60 percent slower. The number of muscle fibers declines by 3 to 5 percent each decade; muscle strength has been reduced by 10 to 30 percent by age sixty. By seventy, the body uses 10 percent fewer calories when at rest; excess calories are spent making fat, which replaces lost muscle. By the same age, nerve signals travel up to 15 percent slower, joints are as much as 30 percent less flexible, and bones are getting brittle. A seventy-year-old man has lost an average of 15 to 20 percent of his bone mass; a woman the same age has lost an average of

25 to 30 percent. By seventy-five, the chest wall has stiffened and lung capacity has shrunk: A man gets 50 percent less oxygen, a woman 29 percent less, than when they were young. Even the kidneys shrink with age.

But take heart. These statistics are for "normal" people, who, in our society, are normally sedentary. About half this normal decline is due to disuse. A moderate, balanced fitness program slows time's clock, as though for each year mere months had passed.

More remarkable still is that time's clock can be reversed, and not only in people as young as fifty but even beginning in the seventies or eighties. Or later: A ninety-year-old can more than double his or her muscle strength. Every item on the aging list can be improved, including breathing and heart function, bone density and organ size, work capacity and mood. Gains earned in a year can shed twenty years. The good news is that aging is reversible: You can go back again.

The bad news is that the gains aren't permanent. Three weeks in bed can age a person the physiological equivalent of thirty years, and even a week of shirking can start to unravel a year's reknitting of bone and sinew.

A fitness program is therefore similar to a diet: When you stop dieting, you regain what you lost; when you stop exercising, you lose what you gained.

A Skeleton in the Closet

I seldom have much trouble getting people started on exercises. The trouble is getting anyone to keep them up. Pain goes, strength returns, they quit. The body can't keep its owner informed of minor developments, such as the insidious and invisible ways in which it's aging.

I keep a little skeleton and some models of human joints in a closet to show injured patients how a body is put together and how they've managed to tear it apart. "Do I really look like that?" they ask,

The Elixir of Youth

Researchers recently reported the discovery of a genuine elixir of youth: a growth hormone that reverses aging. In those who took the drug, bones became denser, muscles stronger, skin thicker, smoother, and more youthful looking. But don't get your hopes up.

The catch to the growth hormone treatment, as discussed in the *New England Journal of Medicine* during the summer of 1990, is that it was tried only with a small group of men who were unusually deficient in their own natural growth hormone. They required three injections a week, at a cost of $14,000 a year. If taken by those who have no growth hormone deficiency, the hormone can cause high blood pressure, diabetes, overgrowth of the face and hands, heart problems, and cancer.

and I say, "Your face is gorgeous, but that's what you're like inside." It took a lesson in anatomy to heal the fencing master and to keep him healed.

This handsome he-man with a swagger that would knock your socks off insisted on fencing with the same vigor that had won him a medal in the Olympics forty years before and had the crippled knees to prove it. Some minutes studying the delicacy of a knee joint — accompanied by my vivid voiceover about what he'd done to his — convinced him to mend his ways and knees. If the skeleton strategy hadn't worked, he would have limped back sooner or later, and I would at least have had a second chance.

I'll get no second chance with you. Although I'll treat you to some drawings of bones and joints for your anatomical education, much of aging happens microscopically, at too small a scale to either see or feel until the damage is done. Yet it's in just this microscopic world, where cells live and work, that lifting a dumbbell or stretching a joint is most exquisitely felt. If exercise weren't felt by the cells, the body wouldn't be renewable, and you could spare yourself the effort to delay its aging.

So let me introduce you to your interior landscape and to the cells that dwell there. I hope the pathos of their little lives will help you persevere.

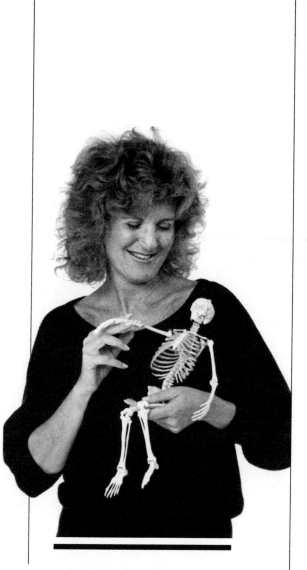

Carol Greenberg with her little skeleton

TWO

The Renewable
Body

C ells come in more varieties than Baskin-Robbins ice cream, and only a few (fat cells, for example) resemble the sedentary and squishy blobs that most of us picture if we think of cells at all. Were you out in the sun today? Pigment makers, like tattoo artists, are now injecting their brown dye into your skin cells through their outstretched tentacles. Did a mosquito bite you? Speckled cells inside your skin are erupting spurts of itching juice. Giant scavengers are creeping toward the bite to engulf germs and fatally digest them. Spidery cells have already begun to reweave the fabric of your skin.

Yes, fabric. Skin, nails, hair, teeth, bones, tendons, ligaments, and the whole mesh of connective tissue that sheaths your muscles and keeps your guts in place are largely materials made *by* cells, not of them. Beneath the single layer of cells that renews your skin's worn surface is a thick-spun felt that, dried and scraped of fat, you'd recognize as leather.

Cells are living, sentient, chemically chatty critters who respond to their environment with remarkable sensitivity and precision. The rest of you is dead. Dead, but renewable.

Bone Builders

Take your buttocks bones. If you lead a sit-down life, they are thickened at the bottom where they press against a chair. That's because their makers, plump but on-the-move cells called osteoblasts ("bone builders"), detect which portions of their product are under pressure and buttress that part to take the extra stress. Pitchers develop tough knobs at the shoulder and elbow where their throwing muscles pull against the bone. Runners get thick legs; farmers get thick hands. I suppose soccer players get thick skulls. The bones of astronauts, however, thin and lighten during every trip into space. Floating in zero gravity doesn't burden bones enough to keep their makers lively.

Bone rebuilding goes on all the time and at such a rate that there's no bone in your body more than ten years old. Right now, in your hands, crews of bone tunnelers called osteoclasts ("bone destroyers") are dissolving new channels in old bone in your fingers. They crawl along, spitting erosive chemicals ahead of them, leaving a cavity in the bone behind them. Into this cavity sprouts a new branch of blood vessel that leaks out plasma to keep the crew supplied with oxygen and food. A crowd of bone builders arrives. They ooze themselves out along the walls of the new channel, secreting a network of flexible fibers that coat it entirely. Crew after crew of builders adds new layers to the tunnel, and over the days, as calcium crystallizes within their handiwork, the layers harden into bone.

My co-author's grandmother was in the habit of breaking apples. She broke them right in half, right into her nineties. Her bone crews built her fingers thick: Tunnelers made more and bigger channels; builders coated them more thickly. Through the complex chemistry of bone stress that isn't yet well understood, crystallization went on at a peppier pace than in those who merely wave their fingers in the air. Those hands were as solid as a rock.

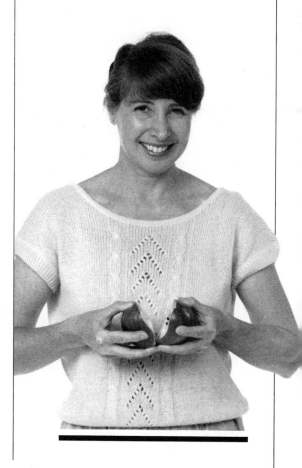

A hint on breaking apples: Choose a small, crisp Mcintosh or cheat, as we did, by making a small cut first!

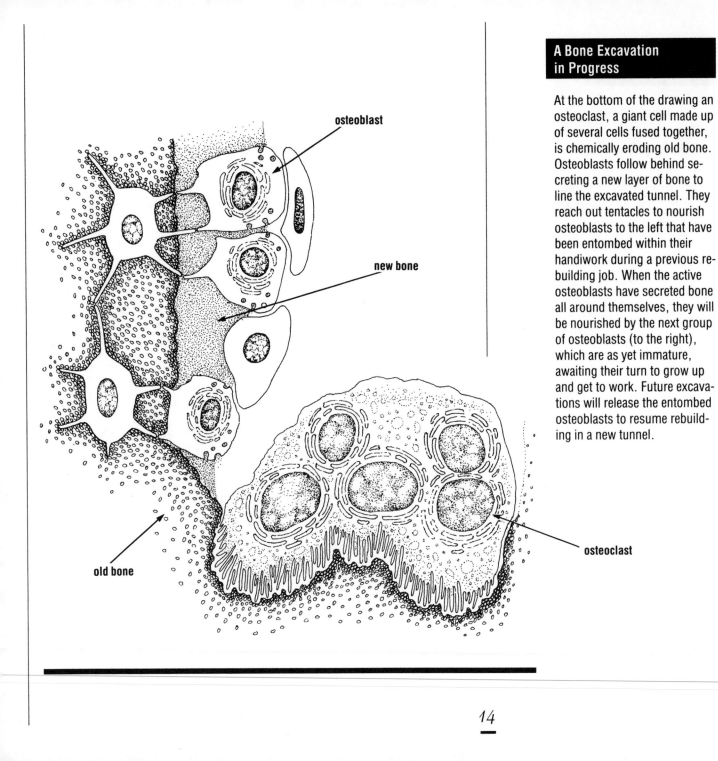

osteoblast

new bone

old bone

osteoclast

A Bone Excavation in Progress

At the bottom of the drawing an osteoclast, a giant cell made up of several cells fused together, is chemically eroding old bone. Osteoblasts follow behind secreting a new layer of bone to line the excavated tunnel. They reach out tentacles to nourish osteoblasts to the left that have been entombed within their handiwork during a previous rebuilding job. When the active osteoblasts have secreted bone all around themselves, they will be nourished by the next group of osteoblasts (to the right), which are as yet immature, awaiting their turn to grow up and get to work. Future excavations will release the entombed osteoblasts to resume rebuilding in a new tunnel.

Scuffing skin, working a muscle, and stretching a tendon are similar to burdening a bone: These actions ask some accommodation of living cells, which, through their changed behavior, reply. The language by which you pose problems and receive solutions is one of chemicals, and very often the opening statement is a declaration of damage. So it is with the signal to build a callous.

Your outer covering (the stuff that peels from sunburned shoulders) is built by a layer of reproducing cells that, as they multiply, squeeze their offspring up toward the surface. For a while, new layers of squeezed-up offspring manufacture the tough fiber called keratin, which is also the main ingredient of hair and fingernails. As the cells near the surface, they die and become the keratin-toughened flakes that you know as dandruff. Under ordinary circumstances, about as many flakes scuff off as new cells are squeezed up, so your skin stays the same thickness from day to day.

When you continually scuff your palm by hoeing the vegetable garden, senescent cells still on their way up to flakiness are damaged. They leak out a chemical that is received by the multiplying cells below and that makes them multiply faster. More new layers are now added than worn off, thickening the skin into a protective callous. Notice that meanwhile your palms hurt: Sometimes you have to suffer a bit to speak in a chemically loud enough voice to rouse your cells to action.

You also have to speak consistently and repeat yourself a lot, just as you might to keep a child at his chores. A day's hoeing may give you blisters but no callouses. Hoeing only on Sundays won't do it, either. Building bodies isn't like building houses, where each new piece of lumber is a permanent addition to the structure. Skin flakes, bone disintegrates, and muscles fall apart if they're not rebuilt continually.

Chemical Conversations

Cells are enclosed in an oily membrane much like the surface of a soap bubble. Studded through this membrane are amazingly complicated protein molecules of hundreds — possibly thousands — of different kinds. Some act as portals through which food molecules are transported into the interior of the cell. Others, called receptors, are shaped to grasp chemical messages in the form of hormones and other molecules secreted by cells elsewhere in the body.

When a receptor is filled by the molecule it's designed to fit, it snaps into a shape that triggers a specific chemical response inside the cell membrane. Sometimes the response is mediated by a protein released by the receptor as it is filled. A manufacturing process may be started up, or a gene that codes for a specific product may be activated. That product may be for the cell's own use, or it may be a chemical reply that, secreted into the bloodstream, is grasped by the receptors of other, distant cells.

The speed and volume of these transmissions are amazing. Blood travels the full circuit of the body in twenty seconds. A single messenger molecule alighting on a receptor can trigger the manufacture of millions of molecules of product in less than a second.

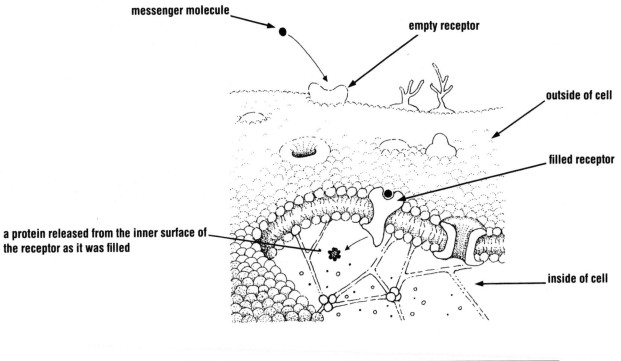

messenger molecule

empty receptor

outside of cell

filled receptor

a protein released from the inner surface of the receptor as it was filled

inside of cell

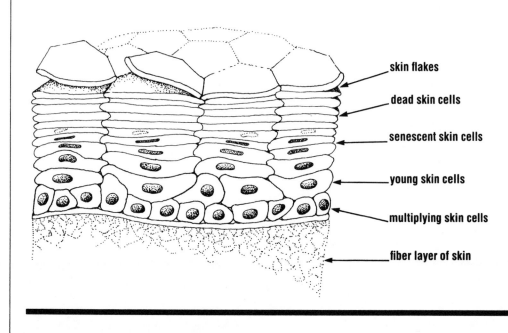

skin flakes

dead skin cells

senescent skin cells

young skin cells

multiplying skin cells

fiber layer of skin

A Small Section of Skin

The layer of stacked cells that constitute your surface is roughly the thickness of skin that peels from a blister. Beneath the surface skin is a much thicker layer made up of a mesh of fibers and containing blood vessels, sensory nerve endings, sweat and oil glands, as well as a padding of fat.

Machinery to Move a Muscle

The muscles that thump your heart or swallow your food are made up of individual cells, each with its own nucleus where it keeps its genes. The muscles that work your skeleton are different. Each is made up of sheaves of muscle fibers (the sheaves are what you see as the stringiness of meat), and each muscle fiber is an elongated group of cells that, merging their surface membranes and leaving their nuclei on the outside, fused when you were an embryo. Most cells can reproduce by duplicating their various internal organs and pinching themselves in two. Cell reproduction is usually also cell rejuvenation: Splitting is like starting all over again. Muscle fibers, however, can't reproduce. Those you were born with were the maximum number you would ever have; some have died in the meantime, and those that remain are now as old as you. The only way to get stronger is to tell the muscle fibers to manufacture more of their internal equipment, the microscopic molecular machinery that pulls your muscles short.

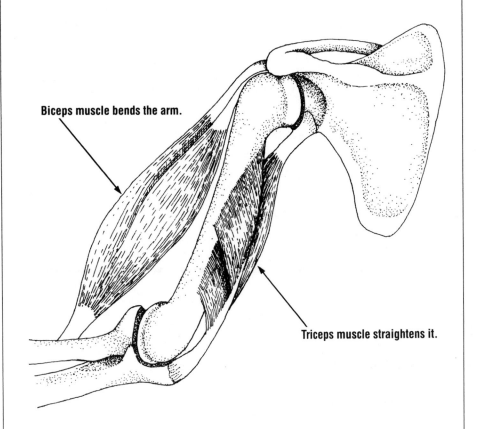

Biceps muscle bends the arm.

Triceps muscle straightens it.

Your arms are engineered to push as well as pull, but muscles only pull. Whether you pull a book from the shelf or push it back again, the action results from muscles pulling. The big biceps in your upper arm shortens to pull the forearm bent. Then an opposite muscle on the underside of your arm shortens to pull the forearm straight. The biceps meanwhile relaxes and lengthens, but there's no force in that.

Minuscule Muscles

Each muscle, such as the spindle-shape biceps, is made up of muscle fibers, each of which is a large group of fused muscle cells whose nuclei lie just beneath the surface of the membrane that encloses them. The fiber appears striped because of the regular arrangement of contractile machinery inside it. The machinery is lengthy assemblies of rod- and tube-shape molecules that slide along one another to shorten like a TV antenna. When you flex your biceps, it is these molecules that make the motion and do the work.

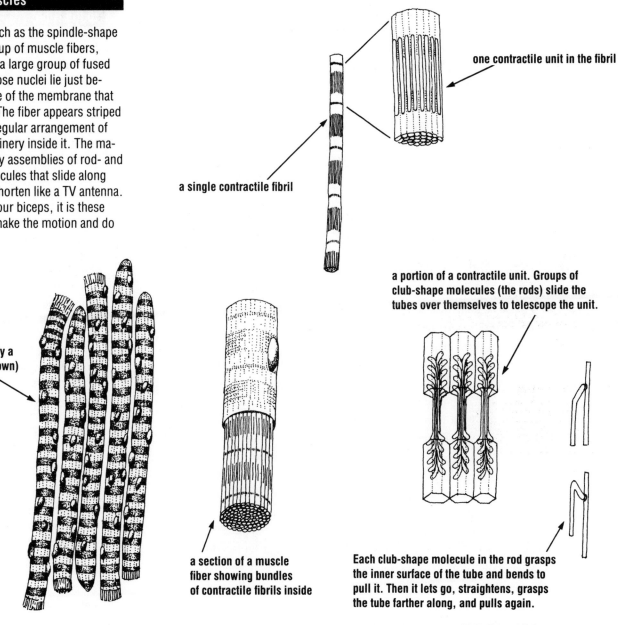

one contractile unit in the fibril

a single contractile fibril

a portion of a contractile unit. Groups of club-shape molecules (the rods) slide the tubes over themselves to telescope the unit.

muscle fibers (only a part of each is shown)

a section of a muscle fiber showing bundles of contractile fibrils inside

Each club-shape molecule in the rod grasps the inner surface of the tube and bends to pull it. Then it lets go, straightens, grasps the tube farther along, and pulls again.

Pulling is done by rod- and tube-shape molecules in telescoping units laid end to end and thickly bundled within the muscle fiber. The bundles stuff the fiber, giving it a meaty texture. At the signal to contract, the rods slide the tubes over themselves, collapsing the whole assembly like a telescope or TV antenna. The collapsing is done by little feet along the rods that yank at the tubes. When a muscle relaxes, the little feet let go and the tubes slide apart again. The feet are fueled — never mind the details — by fat and sugar with the help of oxygen, and the signal to contract is relayed from the brain via neurons (nerve cells), whose branches contact each muscle fiber individually, in synchrony. A whole muscle — a biceps, for example — is made up of hundreds of thousands of muscle fibers all working in unison.

Muscle power is a question of quantity: how many rods and tubes a muscle fiber has. A muscle fiber makes its machinery according to demand.

Always — and this is true of any body molecule — a number of rods and tubes fall apart daily and are replaced, more or less — more if you use the muscle, less if you don't. Each time a muscle fiber is signaled, it receives from its neuron a chemical that not only tells it to contract, but that gives a little kick to its molecular assembly line as well. The less you use a muscle, the less self-repair it does and the smaller and weaker it becomes. A muscle fiber that receives few signals withers and eventually may die.

Lazy movement is not enough to make a muscle stronger. You have to work it. Were you to work an arm unusually hard — lifting heavy tomes rather than lightweight paperbacks — there would be an unusual amount of equipment breakage within the muscle fibers, and they would respond by stepping up production even more than they would from a signal just to twitch. You could feel the damage if you lifted dictionaries for a day: By the next morning your arms would be sore when they moved, the muscles tender to the touch. But were you to lift dictionaries daily, you would end up with strong arms. Less lifting, using lighter weights, would strengthen you more gradually and without noticeable soreness. Imagine hoisting dumbbells three times a week, and you get the idea.

A Fibroblast Ruffling to the Right

Fibroblasts move by ruffling. The ruffles curl up in front and fall back as waves of ripples that gradually subside. Meanwhile, membrane beneath the cell flows forward, moving the fibroblast farther along its way in much the way that tanks move along on caterpillar treads. The pointy extensions to the rear of the cell hold it to the surface as each new ruffle forms, then the points let go and reattach at the next location. Blisters of membrane cover the area of the cell that houses the bulging nucleus. The long spikes are "feelers" by which a fibroblast detects features of its environment — for example, the orientation of the tendon fibers through which it is traveling or a gap where the fabric has been torn.

A tear may be mended or the fabric eased with:

a. twists of tough collagen, which assemble themselves into very long strands
b. snippets of elastin, which form a stretchy mesh
c. enormous water-holding fibers (only part of one is shown here)

These fibers are stored within the cell in membrane-enclosed packages. The packages are delivered to the surface, where they fuse with the cell's outer membrane, open, and release their contents. The fibers are secreted in varying proportions, depending on the type of connective tissue, and are assembled into a mesh outside the cell.

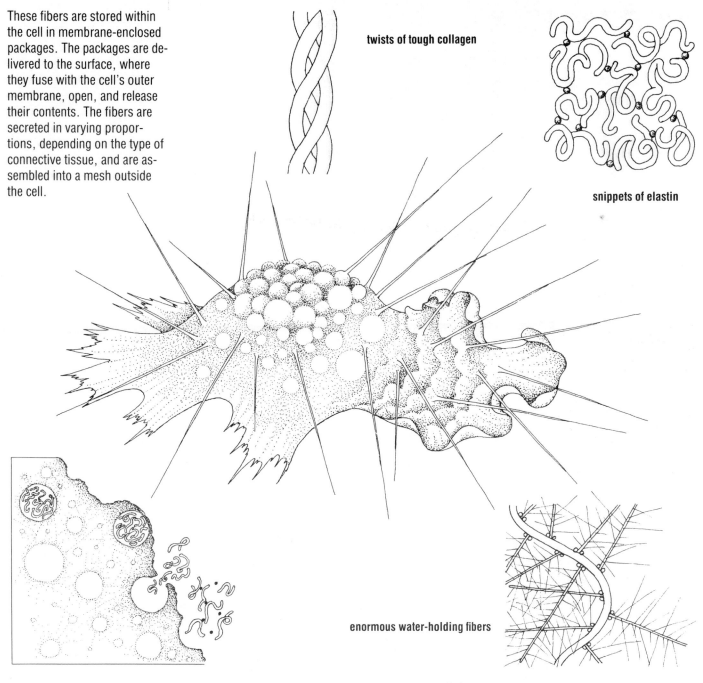

twists of tough collagen

snippets of elastin

enormous water-holding fibers

Besides their active power to contract, muscles have a passive sort of strength: tensile strength, or the ability to resist tearing. As with ropes, the tensile strength of muscles is the greater the thicker they are. The more strands in a rope, the less strain on any one strand when the rope is tensed and the less chance that any strand will break. The same is true of muscles. "Back sprain" most often means back muscle tearing, and thin muscles tear more easily than thick ones.

Muscles are further protected from tearing by the tendon, a material much stronger than raw meat. The tendon sheathes the muscle and attaches it to the bone. The material is the shiny membrane that clothes an uncooked leg of lamb and the gristle that, even when cooked, remains too tough to chew. In a turkey drumstick, those flexible splinters embedded in the meat are the lower ends of tendons that, before its feet were chopped, attached the bird's leg muscles to its toe bones.

Tendons are manufactured by clever, versatile, and mobile cells called fibroblasts ("fiber makers"). Fibroblasts extrude from their innards a variety of fiber molecules, short lengths of which assemble themselves into long strands as they emerge. The fiber that gives a tendon its immense strength is collagen, a triple strand, twisted like a rope, that's glistening and white. Collagen strands in a tendon are laid parallel to one another for maximum strength in the direction of muscle pull.

Fibroblasts weave elasticity into the fabric with short curls of elastin, a molecule that resembles cooked macaroni both in shape and springiness. Elastin curls randomly spot-weld themselves together in a three-dimensional mesh among the strands of collagen. When the mesh is stretched, the macaronis straighten; when it's released, they spring back into curls.

A third fibroblast product is an enormously long, hairy-looking fiber that insinuates itself within the weave, where it attracts and holds water and so plumps up the fabric like a sponge. Fibroblasts also manufacture a sort of universal body glue that cells use for attaching to one another and to the materials that surround them. Just try, for example, to detach the lamb leg's sheathing from its meat!

The sheathing that fibroblasts spin around muscles (and within them, too) is continuous with gristle sheets, which attach muscles to one another, and with the thick bands that attach muscles to bones. The bands are what people usually call tendons, although they're really only the far ends of the entire tendon web. You can feel the great Achilles' tendon at the back of your heel and several tendons behind your knee. Fibroblasts are working there right now.

They work by feel. They creep like amoebas, clutching their handiwork with spiky pseudopods. They orient their innards to match the weave and spin webbing of the proper kind, in the right direction, to maintain the fabric as it wears or mend it if it tears. Are your shoulders stiff from concentrating on the cells' complicated lives? Do that slow shoulder shrug again — up, back, down, and forward. Fibroblasts in the tendons there feel the stretch and spin a little extra fiber to ease the taut bands.

Across the Joint

Lift your index finger. See the tendon in the back of your hand move as you lift? The muscle that contracts to lift the finger is connected by that tendon to your first finger bone; at the other end, the muscle's tendon connects it to an arm bone just below your elbow. Feel the thick tendon in the inside of your elbow? That's the one that connects your biceps to your lower arm; the other end of the biceps is attached at the shoulder. Now straighten your finger and your elbow as far as you can, as if you were pointing an accusing finger at a shameless scoundrel. What prevents the finger from bending toward the sky or the elbow from turning inside out?

The sculpturing of bone ends guides how they move against

each other where they meet, but bands called ligaments, which strap bone to bone across the joint, stop the movement before it's gone too far. Finger joints are just two curved surfaces without any sculpturing to hinder how far a finger bends. If the muscles that lift your fingers were allowed to pull them upright, the force could tear the opposite muscles in your palm, and the finger bones could be pulled right off their perches on the hand. Tendons have to be quite elastic to stretch and rebound as their muscle relaxes and contracts. Ligaments, however, are spun of the toughest collagen fibroblasts can make and are much less generously interwoven with elastin.

Now bend your index finger downward, keeping an eye on the tendon again. You'll notice that it slides over the surface of the finger joint. The joint has to be slippery smooth for the tendon to slide freely, and the bone ends within the knuckle should ideally be cushioned for a frictionless slide as well. I say "ideally" because beyond the age of fifty nothing about joints — neither their smooth, slippery plumpness, nor the elasticity of the tendons that cross them, nor the strength of the

Right Hand, Seen from Above

Only three muscles are shown here: those that lift the thumb and straighten it. If the bones weren't attached by ligaments at their joints, they would be pulled apart by the contracting muscles. The last three fingers are shown with some of the ligaments that prevent that from happening; the index finger is shown with neither muscles nor ligaments. In an actual hand, bands and webs of ligament crisscross the palm and wrist as well to form a complex truss that is strong in all directions.

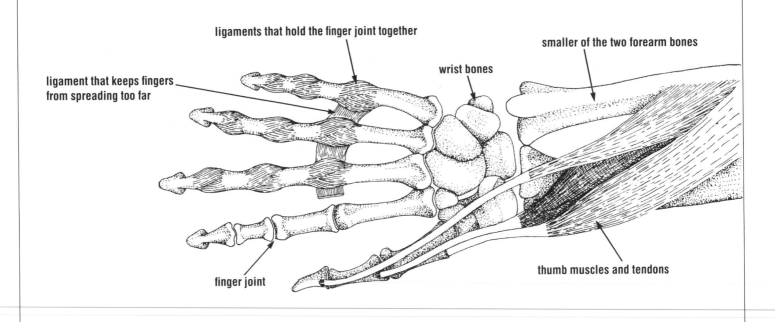

ligaments that hold the finger joint together

ligament that keeps fingers from spreading too far

wrist bones

smaller of the two forearm bones

finger joint

thumb muscles and tendons

muscles that move them, nor the length of the ligaments that strap them, nor the hardness of the bones within them, nor the thickness of the skin that clothes them — is any longer ideal. The fact is, skin cells, muscle fibers, osteoblasts, fibroblasts, and the fibroblast cousins that manufacture cartilage cushioning for joints are all getting older. They haven't lost their skills, but they are slowing down, making less. And their product is deteriorating at a rate they can no longer quite keep up with.

An Older Hand

Picture your parents' hands or your grandparents' hands when you were a child, or if these memories remind you of your own hands now, look at them. Perhaps you can see your veins better than you ever could before. The skin has gotten thinner, and therefore more transparent, because that layer of multiplying cells isn't multiplying so enthusiastically anymore. Pick up a pinch of skin. Maybe it wrinkles and isn't as elastic as it used to be. Fibroblasts, which make the thick felt underlayer of your skin as well as ligaments and tendons, are no longer supplying it with as many stretchy curls or as many of the molecules that plump it up with water.

Their work is also being sabotaged by radicals — free radicals, to use the proper chemical term. Free radicals are fragments of molecules that hunger to become reattached. They're most frequently a by-product of burning — toasting bread, charring steak, caramelizing sugar — but don't think a change in culinary technique will spare you an invasion. Free radicals are common in the air you breathe. They are made in your body, too, and are both a necessary ingredient for, and a by-product of, your body's ordinary chemistry.

The trouble with free radicals is that they glom onto any molecule that accepts them. Fibers accept them very well. Over the years, free radicals attach themselves to fibers and attach the fibers to each other. The effect is something like what happens when you pour glue on cloth. The threads no longer slide freely; the elastic no longer stretches fully: The fabric stiffens.

This happens gradually, over the many years of accumulating free radicals. By the age of fifty, your skin, tendons, and ligaments are stiffening, and there is nothing fibroblasts can do to arrest the saboteurs.

Thinning Pillows

Meanwhile, in the joints, another kind of damage is occurring. Joints are cushioned with cartilage, the white knuckle material that is made of an unusually springy form of collagen by specialized fibroblasts called chondroblasts ("cartilage builders"). Chondroblasts are busiest in babies and young children, where they are fabricating the cartilage scaffolding within which bone builders will work as they add new bone to the growing youngster's skeleton. By the midteens or so, the chondroblasts' masterpiece is finished, and their population has decreased drastically. A few hang out along bone surfaces in case there is a break and their scaffolding services will once again be needed. The others remain in joints repairing cartilage — at a lazy rate.

I don't know why they're lazy. It certainly isn't fair. But it seems to be the rule that chondroblasts don't mend the ordinary wear and tear to joint surfaces as fast as it occurs. Knee joint surfaces gradually roughen and thin from years of squats and jogs and jumps. Cartilage cushions between vertebrae — those notorious disks whose slips and ruptures you've surely heard about — yield to the pressure of gravity and collapse somewhat. Even small actions, like pushing a needle through cloth with the thimble finger, can not only punish a joint with pressure but aggravate it to irrational self-punishment.

Aggravation works this way in any much-used joint: Minor micro-injuries to the cartilage and surrounding tissues call forth troops

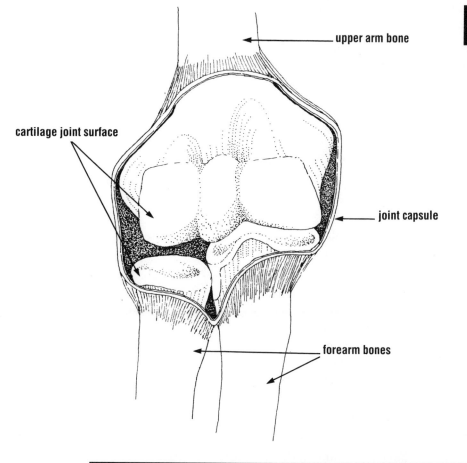

upper arm bone

cartilage joint surface

joint capsule

forearm bones

The whole joint is enclosed by a capsule of ligament that is lined with a thinner, skinlike membrane. The capsule is shown cut open to reveal the joint inside. Fluid within the capsule cushions the bone ends, which are also cushioned by their springy cartilage surface.

whose job is to spray the place with inflammatory chemicals. Inflammatory chemicals, as I'll explain in more detail later, are necessary to healing (they increase the blood supply to the injured area, for example), but they also erode cartilage. The net result of wear and tear to joints is a losing battle in which more cartilage is destroyed than rebuilt.

Between cartilage cushions in a joint is a kind of water pillow: a membrane-enclosed space between the bone ends that is pumped full of fluid. The fluid absorbs pressure like a water bed would do and also lubricates the joint surfaces. Lubrication and cushioning are improved when a joint is in use, for pressure on it squeezes a new supply of fluid from the cartilage, and the water pillow is pumped up to its full capacity. The creakiness of aging joints is due both to their roughened surfaces and to the fact that the cartilage has become too thin to yield as much liquid as it used to.

A Memo to the C.E.O.

This may seem discouraging, but one more point will show you that this lesson in the ways of cells has been steering all along toward an encouraging conclusion.

As communicative as cells are, they rarely talk directly to one another. Muscles don't complain to the joints and tendons that hinder their movements; joints don't cry out to tendons to ease their grip a bit. The complaint department is your brain. All the grumblings of a body now more than half a century old are sent upstairs, straight to the boss.

You, as chief executive officer of your body, can provide the leadership to keep your staff of cells productive even if at times they seem to long for their retirement. Fiber makers will spin more fibers, bone builders will build more bone, muscle fibers will manufacture more muscle machinery, if you only make them move. Believe me, it's true. Exercise and stretch, and you'll even squeeze more juice into your joints.

Sorry about wrinkles. The language of exercise seems not to be spoken in the skin.

THREE

Casual Stretches and Toners

Remember the bendable days of your youth? You were put together with elastic bands then, but your tendons aren't as rubbery anymore. There's nothing you can do about that, because there's no way to get rid of the welds that over the years have stiffened the elastin mesh of your tendons. But suppleness — how far you can move a joint — also depends on the length of the bands that strap your skeleton together and fasten your muscles to your bones. Unlike a wool sweater that got into hot water by mistake, a shrunken band can be eased out to fit its user more loosely.

You've probably noticed shrinkage over the years. It's harder now to reach down to tie your shoes, harder to reach back to clasp your pearls, harder to turn your head to see behind you.

The harder it gets, the less you move. The less you move, the stiffer you get. You're stiffening up all over, and now you know why microscopically: You've told your fibroblasts to rest from their spinning labors.

Remember that those many-armed weavers that make your straps hold on to their handiwork. They learn from the tension of the fibers surrounding them how to pace their production. If a tendon or ligament is slack, they add fewer new units to replace those worn away, so the strap shortens. If the strap is pulled, they splice additional lengths of fiber into the weave, so the fabric lengthens. Therefore the antidote to the increasingly limited range of motion that handicaps so many older people is simply stretching.

A stretch is a slow, gentle movement of a joint that pulls its tendons and ligaments slightly farther than they're used to. Think of a stretch as literally tugging at the arms of fibroblasts, coaxing them to yield those tiny snippets of fiber that will gradually ease the bands that now restrict your movement.

As tendons are stretched, so are the muscles they sheathe. Cramped, tensely telescoped muscle fibers release their grip and extend to their full length. That feels good. Cramped muscles constrict their own blood supply. When you stretch a muscle, you relax it, letting more blood flow and bringing in fresh oxygen. Stretching relieves the achiness you feel after sitting too long in one position or even after lying too long in bed. If you wake up hurting in the morning, stretching will likely ease the pain.

Since worn, complaining joints may begin the sore spiral toward a stiff old age, one would hope that stretching muffles their nagging voices too. It does. Pressure within the joint space works very well to pump up the water bed as you stretch and lubricate the worn joint surfaces. I used to beg my grandmother to stretch and flex her hands to relieve her arthritic knuckles. "Ich kann nicht," she objected, because of course it hurt to do it. The reward of less pain comes after, not during, the stretch; the ultimate reward is less rapid joint deterioration and enough suppleness to do as you wish on your own even when you're truly aged.

In other words, the only way to keep moving is to keep moving.

It's Easier Than You Think

Although suppleness doesn't improve overnight, you'll notice a greater freedom of motion after about two weeks of stretching. It takes several months to become as flexible as the condition of your joints will allow.

You don't have to do all these stretches every day. A few times a week is usually enough. On the other hand, these casual stretches feel really good, are easy to do, and can be done at odd moments —when you're waiting for the toast to pop or for a real person to speak to you on the telephone. How many times a day do you take thirty seconds off to stare at the wall? That's all the time a stretch takes.

All these stretches together take about five minutes, but I wouldn't do them all in a single session. It's too dull and isn't motivated by the discomforts that stretches are meant to relieve. Stretch your neck and shoulders whenever you catch them cramped. Do waist bends, thigh pulls, and calf stretches during commercials or to loosen up after a long commute. Feel free to bend your wrists and twirl your ankles anytime.

I tell my patients to hold each stretch for a count of three and to repeat the motion five times for each joint being stretched, alternating between left and right or back and front. However, stretching is not a sacred rite. I used to tell patients to hold each stretch for a count of ten and repeat it twice. Their boredom with this slow rhythm convinced me to change the pace, and you can change it further any way you please as long as the stretch is slow and held for at least several seconds. What you don't want to do is speed a stretch up to the point where you're jerking or bouncing a joint. Sudden stretches make muscles tighten, not loosen, and so defeat the purpose of the exercise. Rest for a second or two between stretches. Develop your own mental chant to keep the slow, easy beat. Like "Push (or pull) and one and two and three and rest. Rest. Push and one and two and three and rest. Rest." Maybe you can be more poetic, but you get the idea.

The stretches that follow are arranged from head to toe, but a few more rigorous trunk stretches are saved for the routine to be done privately three times a week, as described in the next chapter.

A Head-to-Toe Experiment

After you've learned all the stretches, both the casual ones and those that are included in the thrice-weekly routine, you might try just once doing all of them in order from top to bottom, starting with the neck and ending with the feet. This is the way the yawn and stretch that nature gave us to start our day each morning flows down from the jaw to the fingertips and toes. The experiment can be revealing. When you stretch your neck, then your shoulders, then your wrists and fingers, the flow of relaxation gives a sense of how a body is strung together, how holding the neck stiffly prevents the arms from swinging freely and clenches the hands as well. Moving downward, a stiff back locks hips, locked hips shorten the stride, and a short stride makes people hobble on their feet instead of rolling along from heel to toe.

Pull your head sideways: Hold your head up, with chin tucked and eyes glued to something straight in front of you. Reach your right hand over the top of your head, hold your skull just above your ear and gently pull your head sideways. Count to three, relax, then pull in the other direction with your left hand. Pull each side five times altogether. You should feel the stretch both in the neck and shoulder of the side that's being pulled.

The head pull, combined with the two stretches that follow, can ease a tension headache because that pain, typically in the rear of the head, is caused when cramped neck muscles pinch the blood supply to the back of the neck and the scalp and skull above it.

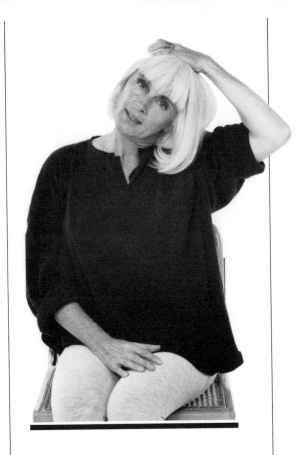

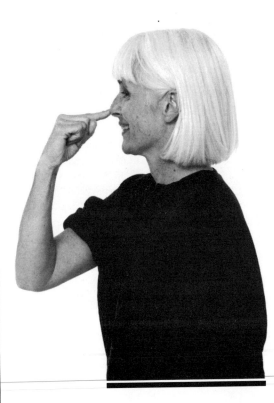

Push your head back: Put your finger on your nose, tuck your chin, and guide your head straight back until your ears are beyond your shoulders — or as near to that goal as you can get. Don't forget to hold, relax, and repeat. You'll feel this one at the base of your neck and in your upper back between the shoulder blades.

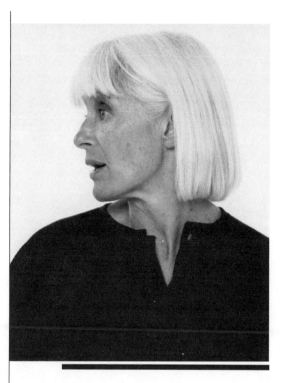

Turn your head from side to side: Tuck your chin. Then slowly turn your head with the aim of getting your chin to point at your shoulder. Turn to one side, then the other, each time counting to three before relaxing and repeating. There's a temptation to also swivel your shoulders, as when trying to see what's going on behind your back, but don't. You should feel this stretch only in your neck, not in your shoulders or rib cage.

Practice this head turn when you're curious to see what's going on behind you. Turn your head first, and swivel the rest of your body only if you still can't see what's happening.

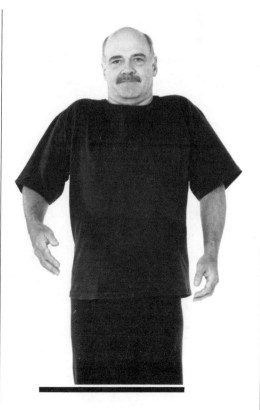

Shrug your shoulders: Sitting or standing, let your arms hang limply at your sides (*not* like my friend here, whose tension was caused more by the camera than by the rigors of this easy stretch). Shrug both shoulders up, back, down, and forward in as large a circle as you can. To give yourself impossible but graphic goals, try to reach your shoulders to your ears as they come up, to touch your shoulder blades together as they come back, to reach your hands to your knees as they come down, and to touch your shoulders to each other as they come forward. Then shrug your shoulders in the opposite direction — up, forward, down, and back. There's no counting or holding for this stretch. You want a slow, continuous movement.

You could also shrug one shoulder at a time. Tasks like embroidering or addressing envelopes by hand often tax the shoulder on the working side (left or right, depending on your handedness). A one-shoulder shrug is a great relief.

33

Here's a variation of the shoulder shrug that stretches ligaments and muscles in the upper chest as well as in the shoulders. Bend your arms like chicken wings; your hands should be up in your armpits. Now flap in a large, slow circle.

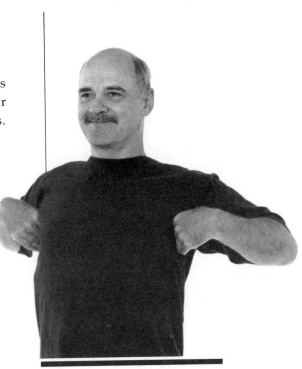

Push your elbow over your shoulder: This stretch is a little hard to get the knack of. Hang one arm over your shoulder, with the hand dangling down behind your neck. With your other hand, push the elbow back until you feel the stretch under the pushed arm and along that side of your chest. Count to three, and repeat the usual number of times.

Hint: The stretch, properly done, should enable you to scratch a mosquito bite on the upper edge of your shoulder blade.

Pull your elbow across your chest: Crook one arm in front of you; you should be staring at your fist. Hold the crooked elbow with your other hand and pull it across your chest. You'll feel this stretch behind, in the shoulder blade of the arm you're pulling. Count to three, let your elbow go, and repeat the pull using the opposite arm. Do it five times per side, ten times altogether.

Try this stretch to relieve stiffness from holding a steering wheel, typing, knitting, or even holding a "can't put it down" novel.

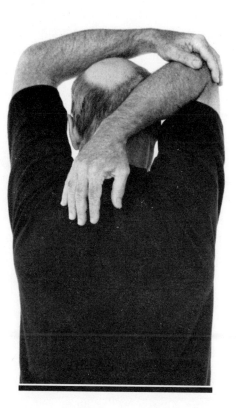

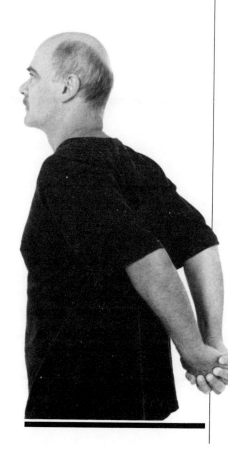

Lift your clasped hands behind your back: Let your arms hang and clasp your hands behind your back. Pull your shoulder blades together, then lift your clasped hands. Hold for a count of three, relax, repeat five times. You'll feel the stretch in the front this time, up near your collar bone.

Bend your wrists: Use one hand to push the other back as far as the wrist will bend, then forward. There's no particular count or number of repeats for this one; you'll want to do it often if you type a lot.

Flapping the hands with wrists loose relaxes cramped fingers as well as wrists.

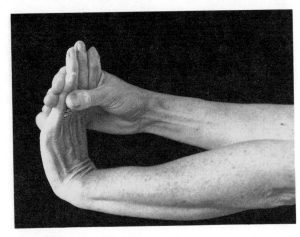 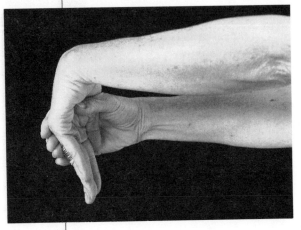

Stretch and flex your fingers: Spread and straighten your fingers as far as they'll go, then flex them into a fist. This will feel particularly good after you've been writing or driving for too long without a break. Again, there's no reason to count this stretch.

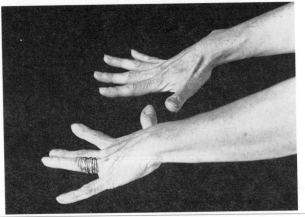 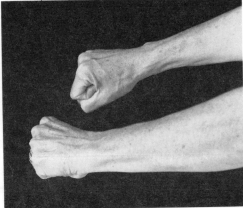

Bend at the waist: Put your hands on your hips and bend slowly sideways as though trying to touch your elbow to your knee, first in one direction, then the other, each time far enough to feel the stretch in your waist. Hold each stretch for a count of three, and do each side five times.

Hip-wiggling wouldn't hurt, either, and you can do it while washing dishes. Shift your weight onto one foot, and stick that hip out sideways. Shift to the other foot, and stick that hip out. Finish the dishes, turn on some music, add a step to each shift, and you're dancing!

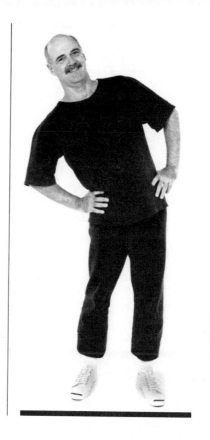

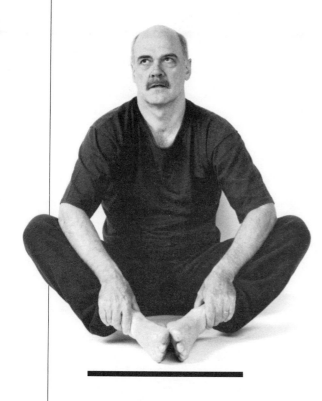

Stretch your groin: This stretch is for when you're sitting on the sofa munching pretzels, watching the news. Budge your behind into the sofa so that you can lean your back against it. Sit with your knees bent and the soles of your feet together — or as close to it as stiffness will allow. Grasp your ankles, put your elbows on your thighs, and gently press your legs down. You're sure to feel this stretch — right in the groin where the inner muscles of your thighs attach.

It may be hard at first to hold this stretch as long or repeat it as many times as usual. Still, aim for a hold of three, a repeat of five.

Another, even less formal way to stretch the groin is to sit for a few minutes Indian style, the way you did once upon a time in nursery school. Sitting with an ankle cocked on the knee in the manner of a man at ease stretches bands in the side of the hip.

Stretch your thighs: Do this thigh stretch standing on one leg and holding the edge of a table, counter, or the back of a sturdy chair for support. Reach your free hand behind you and grab the opposite foot. Stand straight, and pull the foot up until the knee of that leg is next to the other one. You'll feel it in the front of your thigh. It's nasty, but you can see why you need it. You may be too stiff to even reach your ankle with the opposite hand. In that case, use the hand on the same side until you've become loose enough to stretch your thigh the harder way.

In these days of jogging suits and public warm-ups, thigh stretches while filling up on gas aren't out of place provided you're wearing pants, not a skirt. You'll appreciate how nicely they alleviate tightness in the leg that's pressed for hours to the accelerator on a long trip. Use the roof of the car for support.

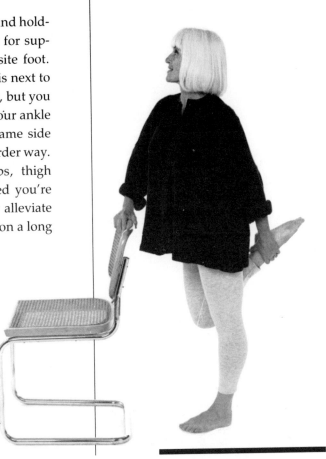

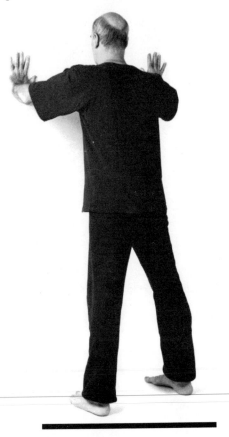

Stretch your calves: Lean with your hands against the wall; your feet should be about eight inches apart and about thirty inches from the wall. Keep your back straight and stand pigeon-toed. Now bend your elbows until you feel your calf muscles stretch. Count to three before straightening your arms again, and repeat five times.

This stretch feels especially good to women who have shortened their calf muscles too much by wearing high heels.

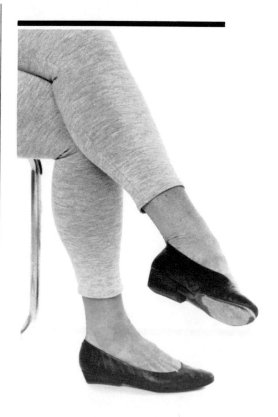

Twirl your ankles: While sitting in a chair, straighten one leg and slowly circle the foot. Change legs to twirl the other ankle. You'll feel this stretch in your shin as well as in your calf and ankle joint. You don't have to count twirls; just do them for comfort.

This is the least obtrusive of the stretches that are helpful to those who travel a lot in planes. The enormous discomfort suffered by frequent travelers and long-distance vacationers calls for all the stretches you can possibly do while in the torture chamber of an airplane seat or in the aisles between feeding times.

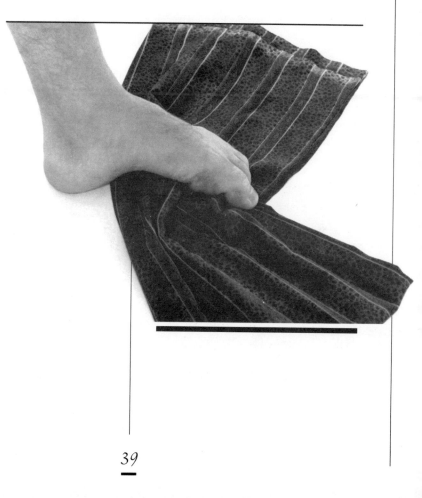

Curl your toes: Sit barefoot in the kitchen or bathroom (where there isn't any carpet) and put a small towel on the floor in front of you. Try, by curling your toes over the towel edge again and again, to scrunch it up underneath your foot.

After you've practiced this curling motion a few times, you can dispense with the towel and do the stretch anywhere, such as under your desk with your shoes slipped off. You'll feel this stretch in the arch of your foot, and you'll like the feeling a lot. It's great for aching feet after you've been standing all day.

The Difference Between Lax and Relax

A resting muscle is relaxed, but not flaccid. Here and there throughout each muscle fiber some telescoping units are contracting somewhat, giving the muscle the firmness called tone. Tone readies muscles to escalate their effort in a split second. When a muscle has poor tone — too little machinery contracting — any sudden call to action catches it off guard and easily throws it into spasm. That's what happened to my patient who was felled to the kitchen floor by picking up a can of stewed tomatoes. Her lax muscles, overstretched by the bend, recoiled defensively and tightened into knots of painful contraction.

Isometrics, exercises that require pressure but no motion, restore and maintain muscle tone. Mushy tummies and flabby backsides lack tone. Your neck muscles may not sag, but they are probably less firm than they could be, and they could knot at the jerk of a head. Scrawny chests reveal that the muscles there are drooping.

These isometric exercises are so unobtrusive that they can be done publicly yet secretly. Some are invisible; others so resemble ordinary poses that, at most, people will think you hurt somewhere. In some you just tighten a set of muscles, as in tightening your abdomen. No one can see you do that. In others you oppose the pressure of two sets of muscles, as in resisting the pressure of your hand pushing against your head.

Unless I tell you otherwise for a particular isometric, hold the tension for the count of three. Relax. Tighten again. The number of times is up to you, but five repeats per exercise is a minimum, and a daily dose is necessary for firmness you can notice.

The Toners

Pull and push your head: These three isometrics tone neck muscles. Neither your head nor the hands that press against it should move during the exercise. You want force, not action.

First, with elbows out, clasp both hands behind your head. Pull forward with your hands as you push backward with your head.

The second takes more time and may make people think you have a headache. Hold your head straight and still, as though you're trying to impress someone with your dignity. Press the palm of one

hand to your forehead and resist the pressure with your head. Then do the same thing with your palm pressed to the back of your skull.

Tone the muscles in the sides of your neck by pressing your palm against your skull just above your ear, first one side, then the other.

In combination with neck stretches, these head presses are particularly helpful to people who have that common affliction of aging, arthritis of the neck vertebrae; in fact, the first press does double duty as both a stretcher and a toner.

Push your palms against each other: This toner firms the muscles of the upper chest. With elbows lifted and hands clasped, push your palms against each other.

Don't expect this exercise to lift sagging breasts, but firmer muscles will help to fill in a scrawny chest.

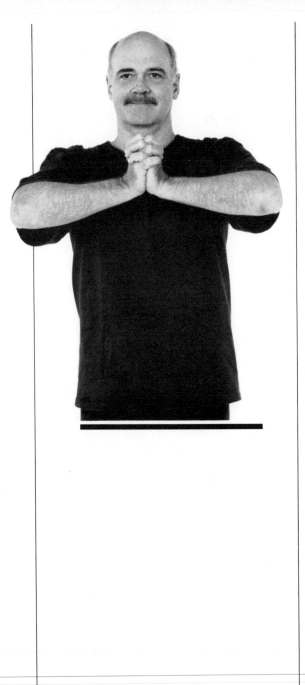

Tighten your belly: Your abdomen is crisscrossed with bands of belly muscle that, when taut, act as a girdle to hold in your guts and take the strain off your back. However, any bulge of fat you may have lies on top of the muscles, not below them, so a tighter muscle girdle won't help you there.

First, tighten your abdominal muscles as though tensing to push a great weight. You'll feel like holding your breath, but I want you to breathe three times in and three times out while holding your belly taut. You can do this toner while you walk.

Then work a somewhat different set of abdominal muscles by pulling your belly in as though to touch your belly button to your spine. Hold this tension as long as concentration allows, and tense again whenever you notice that your belly's slack. It could become a habit!

Buttocks firmers: While standing, tighten your buttocks as hard as you can, as though you had to crack a walnut between them. Hold them tight for several seconds before relaxing and repeating.

While sitting, do the same exercise — but not if anyone's watching. Tightening and relaxing your buttocks when you're sitting bounces you up and down in your chair and looks mighty peculiar.

Now that you've read through the instructions for these twenty or so stretchers and toners, you may feel there are too many to memorize. Maybe that's so in a word-for-word sense, but memorizing exercises is something like memorizing how to tie a shoelace or drive a car. At first you have to think out each move; you have to remain aware of what you're doing every second. But after a while, memory moves to another part of the brain, where skills are put on automatic pilot. You no longer have to think of which gear is which, what lace goes where, or how to hold your head while stretching.

To get to that level of skill — to go on automatic pilot — give yourself a crash course by doing all these moves every day, by the book, for two weeks, according to a schedule. Yes, take the book with you if you work; it's not heavy, and all you need as a reminder is a quick glance at the picture for the exercise you've scheduled. The schedule should be tailored to your day's routine. If you drive through traffic, you might do the neck exercises while waiting for lights to change. What's done sitting down can be done at a desk, maybe during telephone calls. There's probably some time during the day when you're standing around, waiting for something to happen, such as for the meal to cook. Plan to do standing exercises then.

At the end of the two weeks, the moves will have become automatic as well as integrated into your way of life. What's more, some muscles will be noticeably firmer, and most joints will move more freely.

This first step up from the double jeopardy of stiffness and laxness is a prerequisite for starting the ten-minute workout that comes next. You can read about it now, of course, but firm some sags and limber up some joints before adding these more formal exercises to your age-delay routine.

Sphincter Squeezers

There's an interior muscle that, when it becomes lax, causes one of the most embarrassing and disabling afflictions of age: pants wetting. The doughnut-shape muscle that tightens to prevent urine from leaking out of the bladder is called a sphincter, and it is supposed to be tight enough to keep the opening shut against such pressures as laughing or coughing. It needs good tone to do that, and isometric exercises give it the necessary firmness.

This invisible isometric is especially for women, who leak urine more often than men as they get older. It can be used as a preventive or as a cure. Just squeeze your sphincter shut as though to hold in your urine and keep it tight for three seconds. Ten repeats should work as a preventive. For a cure, aim for fifty to a hundred sphincter squeezes a day.

It's very effective to do the squeezes while urinating. Let some urine out, then try to stop the flow for a count of three; repeat the spurt and squeeze until your bladder is empty.

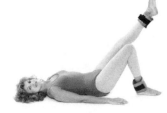

Ten Minutes, Three Times a Week

M ost people like exercise routines about as much as they like to floss their teeth — not much. If they persist, it's on the theory that they're better off groaning figuratively three times a week than groaning literally every time they struggle from a chair. They're right, of course: Body maintenance is a necessary chore.

But surprise! There are no groaners in this routine. These exercises are *easy*! There are only eleven of them. And — this is the best part — they combine stretching with strengthening so that in just weeks you'll feel a new litheness and vigor you may not have known for years. Six months from now, loads will seem lighter, distances shorter, and you'll experience the smug delight of being able to do what others your age can't.

One exercise is an isometric that firms the lower back. Four are trunk stretches that loosen hips and the vertebral joints of your spine. I grouped these five exercises with half a dozen strengtheners partly out of the kindness of my heart. They demand that you descend to the floor, and since you have to be there for leg-strengthening exercises anyway, I thought you might appreciate a single descent.

The strengthening exercises are weight training: muscle workouts that are done by lifting legs or arms weighted with sand or iron. An added benefit of grouping trunk stretches with strengtheners is that if you do everything in the order I've described, your muscles will be prepared for the work they're asked to do. I don't want your back to knot. I don't want you too stiff and sore tomorrow to enjoy your day.

Strength Three Ways

Why get stronger? Not, I hope, because you'd like people to admire your muscles; this isn't a course in body building. Body building involves what seems to me a vain concern with every possible bump of muscle, even those obscure ones that can arise like mushrooms among the ribs.

I care about your *big* muscles, the ones that lift and lug and get you where you're going. I want you to be able to do what you want to do and need to do with ease, without injury. There are triumphant psychological side effects to being strong that I can, and will, wax lyrical about. But let's be medical first.

The greater force that a strong muscle can exert is only one kind of strength. As muscles thicken with weight training, their tensile

Studies in Strength

Recent studies are piling up proof that strengthening exercises work at any age. One study, done as part of a large project on the effects of aging at Tufts University, has found that the loss of muscle mass, once thought to be irreversible, isn't so at all. The subjects were men and women from sixty to ninety-six who underwent a two-month strengthening regime. Those in their sixties and seventies increased their strength by 200 percent; their muscles increased in size by 15 percent. Even subjects in their nineties experienced 180 percent gain in strength, and their muscles grew by 12 percent.

Another study, at the Andrus Gerontology Center at the University of Southern California, Los Angeles, found that men and women from sixty-four to eighty-four who worked out with weights got denser bones as well as stronger muscles. Men benefited the most, but women, in whom osteoporosis is both more common and more severe, enjoyed some improvement too.

strength increases too. The muscle tears less easily, and the joint the muscle spans is also protected. Think of a muscle as a spring on a screen door: the device attached to the door and door frame that works the hinge. You can imagine wrenching a door off its hinges by pushing it too far. Strong springs prevent wrenched hinges; strong muscles at least help to prevent tears to the various soft tissues of a joint.

The second medical reason for strengthening muscles involves blood supply. Oxygen and nutrients dissolved in blood plasma reach muscles through capillaries, vessels so small that red blood cells must squeeze through them single file. A capillary is formed of pancake-shape cells that, curled like crepes, enfold the space inside. These cells divide to form new capillary branches as they're needed, such as when bone building crews need feeding inside a newly excavated tunnel. Red meat gets its ruddy tone from the blood of countless capillaries that penetrate its zillion muscle fibers. But, as with bone, capillaries sprout where the action is: A weak muscle is poorly supplied with the oxygen it needs to do its work.

When you try to work weak muscles, they tire quickly. They feel limp and shaky; they ache urgently for rest. Finally, they collapse. If they're in an arm, the arm drops; if they're in your legs, you drop. With luck into an armchair. I'm sure you know the feeling.

That exhaustion has come about because, as muscle fibers run out of oxygen to extract energy from their store of fat and sugar, they must rely solely on the primitive and inefficient energizing chemistry of fermentation. Fermentation is how bacteria get energy from milk. The sourness of milk after bacteria have finished feeding is a waste product of fermentation called lactic acid. Lactic acid, accumulating in muscles to toxic levels, is what forces them to sourly give out.

Over time, working a muscle attracts more capillaries to it and so brings in more oxygen. A well-supplied limb gains the strength of endurance. You're sure to enjoy raking leaves without your arms giving out, but there's medical significance to increased endurance too. Limbs that give up quickly cause many of the accidents of everyday life, from dropping pots of soup to stumbling over steps.

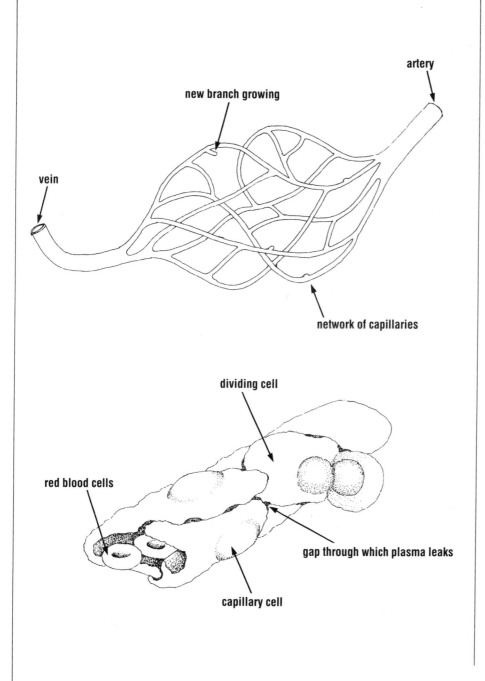

artery

new branch growing

vein

network of capillaries

dividing cell

red blood cells

gap through which plasma leaks

capillary cell

The Smallest Blood Vessels

Blood arriving through an artery from the heart makes its way through a network of capillaries before returning through a vein to the heart. The branchier the network, the better the supply of blood and the more oxygen the muscles receive.

Under greater magnification, each capillary is seen to be formed by flat cells that resemble pancakes — or, because of their large nuclei, fried eggs. Two red blood cells are coming through to the left. To the right, a capillary cell is dividing. Offspring will continue to divide to start a new branch of the capillary. Plasma carrying nutrients as well as oxygen leaks out into the neighborhood through gaps between the ill-fitting capillary cells.

Osteoporosis

Calcium is used for many jobs in the body, not only for hardening bone. In our youth, calcium is dissolved from our bones to be used for other purposes at about the same rate that it is redeposited. As we age, the equation may change: More calcium may come out of our bones than goes back in. As the bones lose the calcium that hardens them, they become porous and brittle. The resulting condition, called osteoporosis, is the cause of most hip fractures. The hunched upper back and noticeable shrinkage of some elderly people come from hairline fractures in their brittle vertebrae.

Osteoporosis is more common in women than in men and is accelerated by the loss of the hormone estrogen when the ovaries cease to function at menopause. One therapy, therefore, is estrogen replacement. Extra calcium in the diet may or may not help; some studies say yes, some say no, but calcium tablets or a diet high in calcium is often prescribed just in case. A helpful drug called Etidronate, now in the last stages of testing in this country, may soon become available. It increases bone density in vertebrae and so prevents hairline fractures in the back. It has no effect on the leg and hip bones.

Walking does. At any age, for both sexes, exercise remains the basic therapy for increasing bone density everywhere in the body.

The third kind of strength is skeletal. Strong muscles heartily tax the bones they pull at, and osteoblasts meet the challenge by making denser bones. The medical advantage is obvious: Dense bones are hard to break.

A Mini-Gym for Over-Fifties

The six weight training exercises here are for the large muscles of the limbs, the beef you need for an active life. They require a pair of iron dumbbells to hold in your hands and a pair of sand-filled ankle weights that wrap around your ankles with Velcro straps.

Both are available in sporting goods stores in various weights, starting at a pound apiece. That doesn't seem like much, but for people who have become very weak from inactivity, even the weight of their own limbs is difficult enough to lift, and I have sometimes started such patients' strengthening with no additional burden at all. Go to a store and try out the weights. Choose 1, 2, 3, or more pounds, depending on which is less than fun to lift but not exhausting, either. If you're not sure, make your mistake on the light side. As you get stronger, use increasingly heavier weights — up to 5 pounds for a woman, 10 pounds for a man.

The only other "equipment" you need to get started is a sturdy, armless chair and a pad to lie on. You'll be lying on the floor, not on a springy bed or soft couch that can't support your back. The pad can be a folded blanket. It doesn't have to be very big; mostly it's the base of the spine that objects to being pressed to a hard floor. If you'd rather go pro, you can buy a small, lightweight exercise pad at the sporting goods store.

Set up your exercise area this way: Roll out the pad in an open, uncluttered space. Put the sturdy chair nearby; position it so that you can sit in it for sitting exercises and hold on to its back during standing exercises. Lay the dumbbells by the chair and the ankle weights by the pad. That's it, a mini-gym for over-fifties.

The routine is arranged so that you don't have to leap up and down from floor to feet and back again. There's nothing athletic here; I mean this routine to be sedate. It's arranged by posture: first, a group of exercises done lying on your back, then onto all fours, up into a chair, and finally standing. When you're finished, you're in a position to walk away from the whole thing and enjoy the rest of your day.

How you lie down is very important, because if you're not snug to the pad you could hurt your back. Lie down with your knees up; press the small of your back to the floor (you can also support the small of your back with a small folded towel placed under it). Tighten your belly: That holds your backbone in place. Each time you finish a floor exercise, check that your back is pressed down and your belly tight, ready to start the next one.

Move slowly and deliberately. If the routine takes less than ten minutes, you've rushed it. I suggest that all the stretches (except the first one, which is a longish stretch for stiff hips) be held for a count of three and repeated five times per side with a rest between each repeat. But, as with casual stretches, you can alter the rhythm to suit yourself as long as you don't jerk your joints or cheat on the total time the tendons and ligaments are stretched. Do strengthening exercises at the same slow speed but more times: ten times per leg, twenty times per arm.

I've noticed two things about weight training. First, these exercises are tiring; few of my patients can do their full quota in the beginning. That's all right; better to go slow and build up gradually. Second, I count faster when doing strengthening exercises than when doing stretches. I don't mean that you *should* count faster; it seems that the tendency to cheat on the length of the effort is greater for the hard work of weight training than for the considerable pleasure of stretching. I didn't notice this until my co-author caught me when we were timing the routine. Perhaps you have some "co-author" in your life who, like mine, has a cod's eye for accuracy.

The Routine

Roll your hips sideways: This is a stretch for hip ligaments, which are often obstinately tight. Move both knees together sideways until they touch the floor. Keep your shoulders flat during the roll: Only the lower half of your body should move, and you should feel the stretch below your waist at your hip and the base of your spine. Roll alternately right and left, and hold this stretch longer, for a count of five, before relaxing. Repeat five times per side.

Cock one leg over the other and lift them both: Cock an ankle over your bent knee. Then move both legs up toward your chest until you feel the stretch in the buttock muscles behind the thigh of the cocked leg and in that hip. Be gentle to yourself — you have weeks in which to ease your tightness gradually. Start with fewer than the usual five lifts per leg but aim for that total, holding each stretch for a count of three.

Straighten your leg: This exercise stretches the great hamstring muscle that spans all the way from the buttocks to the knee. Clasp both hands behind one thigh to support the weight of your leg. Now straighten that leg (or try to). Yes, it hurts. Hamstring muscles and the ligaments back there tend to be exceptionally tight. Alternate legs, and try for five stretches each.

Push and pull your knee: This is an isometric exercise that firms the muscles of the lower back. You must do this toner and the next stretcher to ready your back for the strengtheners that follow.

Lift one knee and push against it with both hands while resisting the pressure with your leg.

Then reverse the action: Clasp both hands in front of your knee and pull, resisting the pressure with your leg. Repeat with the other leg. Don't cheat on the arithmetic — that's five pushes, five pulls, per leg, for a total of twenty.

Pull your knee to your shoulder: Clasp your hands behind one knee and pull it straight back toward the shoulder on the same side. You'll feel the stretch in the muscles of your lower back. Repeat five times per leg, ten knee pulls altogether. (If doing one leg at a time is comfortable, you could try pulling both knees at once to cut the total number of stretches in half.)

Now you're ready for the first strengthening exercise. Sit up for a moment and strap your ankle weights on.

Lift your weighted leg: With your ankle weights on, lie down again, but this time lay one leg out straight instead of bent. Lift that leg until both your knees are level, hold it there for a count of three, let it down again, and relax. Alternate legs to give them a rest between lifts.

Although the aim is to repeat this lift ten times for each leg — twenty times altogether — you may find that number of lifts much too tiring at first. Both your thigh and back muscles are involved, and the ankle weight adds to what is already the heavy burden of a whole leg. Gradually increase the number of lifts from two or three to the total of ten as your muscles get stronger.

The reward for completing this exercise is that you finally get to turn over. Leave the ankle weights on, though. They won't be in your way for the next exercises, and you'll need them again soon.

Arch your back up, then down: Now turn over onto your hands and knees. Bend your head down, tuck your rump in, suck in your belly, and arch your back like a cat. Hold the arch for a count of three, then slowly arch in the opposite direction with your head and rump up and your back slumped down.

This stretch, repeated five times up and five times down, makes your whole back more supple and — congratulations! — you may now get off the floor and sit in the chair.

Bend your weighted arm: Sit in the chair with your back snugged into it. Pick up your dumbbells, one in each hand. Let your arms rest by your sides, then bend one arm at a time to bring the dumbbell up level with your shoulder and let it down again. Hefting weights with the big biceps muscle on your upper arm isn't as tiring as hefting weights with your legs, so aim for twenty bends per arm. Rest as often as you need to. As you get stronger, you may want to cut the total time in half by bending both arms at once.

Lift your weighted arm sideways: Hold the dumbbells with your palms facing in against your thighs. Slowly lift one arm sideways to the level of your shoulders. Most people tend to shrug their shoulders as they do this lift, but don't. Keep your shoulders down. That way just the right muscles — at the side of the upper arm — get strengthened, and you don't risk cramping your neck. Again, try for ten lifts, a rest, and another ten for a total of twenty lifts per arm. If it's not too tiring to lift both arms at once, as in the photograph, by all means do so.

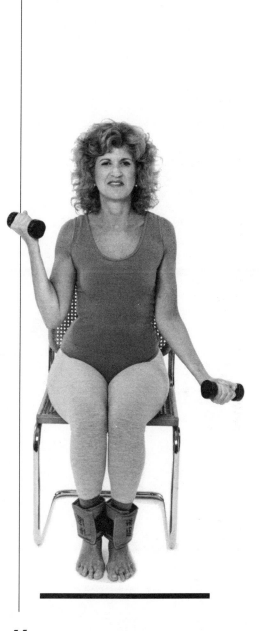

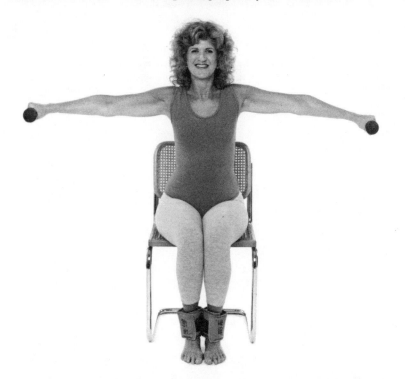

Lift your weighted leg sideways: Now you can stand up, do the last ankle weight exercise, and be done with the sandbags.

Hold on to the back of the chair for support. Keep your abdomen and buttocks tightened. Lift one leg sideways, doing your best to keep the rest of your body straight and still. It's not so easy, and not pain-less either, but aim in the course of a month or so for ten sideways lifts per leg.

Take off your ankle weights if you wish; your legs are done!

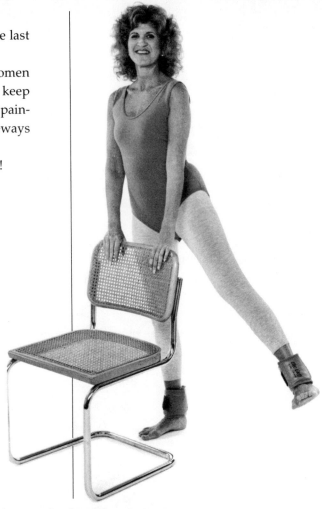

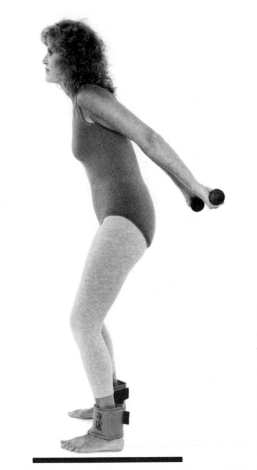

Lift your weighted arms backward: For this exercise, it's important that you stand with your knees slightly bent to prevent strain to your back. Put yourself into a partial crouch, as if you were pretending to be an ape. In this chimp posture, with your arms straight and your palms facing back, lift the dumbbells as high behind you as is comfortable. I guarantee this won't be very far at first, and you'll feel the strain in the triceps muscle under your upper arm. The aim is ten lifts, but don't push it.

If you want to reduce your thrice-weekly routine to exactly ten exercises — and to less than ten minutes — you could strengthen the same arm muscles in a casual way. When you're sitting, place your palms flat on the seat and push down to lift your own weight up. You needn't lift your body clear up in the air; just getting the weight off your buttocks is exercise enough.

After the Work Is Over

And that's it. You can stash your dumbbells and ankle weights, roll up your pad, and get on with other things. Meanwhile, your muscles will be busy building themselves.

A workout is only the beginning of the muscle-building process. Over the next day or so, the muscle fibers you've worked do the actual building of rods and tubes that gradually add bulk. That's nice, because your few minutes of effort are repaid by their many hours of labor.

But don't forget that even as your muscles manufacture new telescoping units, old ones fall apart. The bottom line is that if you do your weight routine just once a week, you will have lost by Thursday what you gained on Monday. You have to do it three times weekly, say, on Monday, Wednesday, and Friday.

So much for scolding; I promised to wax lyrical.

There must be some time you can remember when you were flooded with happiness: a baby born, a wish come true, an effort stunningly rewarded. That flood of joy involves actual substances, especially a group of opiates called endorphins, which are similar to the opium of poppies, and to morphine, which is made from opium. This endogenous joy juice is released within the brain to soothe and celebrate. It causes the euphoria of the runner's "high" and the ascetic's ecstasy. It seems to mediate the general daily cheerfulness of a life well lived. Endorphins are also remarkably effective painkillers.

In large doses, endorphins appear to be the body's way of keeping spirits up and pain at bay during heroic effort. Spurts of these opiates keep athletes going when it seems they ought to drop. Small doses, though, are given as general encouragement during physical and intellectual labor and as a reward for work well done. Even working with your dumbbells may give you an extra drop or two of pleasure. Most important to advocates of exercise, the "background" level of endorphins seems to rise as people improve their physical competence and their level of activity. Exercise has been used for some years now to relieve depression, and people who exercise for other reasons also brighten, often much to their surprise.

When endorphins were first discovered, scientists hoped they had at last found a drug to soothe distress and pain as powerfully as morphine but without addiction. That didn't turn out to be the case. Endorphins are addictive, and wisely so: The best way to satisfy a craving for the body's native joy juice is to repeat the fine achievement that earned a dose before, so endorphins also comprise a self-motivating system.

Work hard, dear reader, and you may become addicted to this exercise routine!

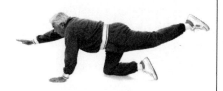

FIVE

A Short Course for Back and Belly

I f you're an average American, you stand better than a fifty-fifty chance of suffering at least one episode of back pain at some time during your life. And, the statistics and my own experience say, the cause of your pain will most likely be back and belly muscles too weak for the strains of everyday life. What's more, if you do nothing to strengthen your trunk after that first back attack, you're more than likely to join the crowd that suffers from chronic backache. Some proportion will fare worse, with serious damage to disks and spinal nerves.

I'll give you an example.

Years ago, when I first opened my practice as a specialist in sports injuries, a young graduate student limped into my office, pale with pain and study. He was no athlete. His back muscles were so meager they couldn't withstand the force of gravity pressing his vertebrae together while he bent over his books. His case history, in brief, was that he had ruptured several disks in his lower back while writing a thesis in sociology and had had to undergo, at the age of twenty-six, spinal fusion surgery. He was a lesson I'll never forget: Neither age nor athletics can beat sheer weakness as the major cause of back problems. That's why I feel no guilt at all instructing even my literary agent to spend minutes every morning looking like a setter flushing birds.

Certainly some back injuries are caused by legitimate accidents: Car crashes and falling headlong down the fire stairs come to mind. But what about the much more usual incidents — teeing off, bending down, lifting pots, digging holes — that are the back-crippling accidents of everyday life? If I've heard it once, I've heard it a thousand times: "I don't understand it. All I did was reach for my hat on the closet shelf (or pick up the suitcase, or hang the picture, or slam the car trunk)." People don't like to blame backaches on themselves.

Psychologists have been overly obliging in this respect. They have ascribed back muscle spasm to work-related stress and marital tensions and have suggested that the pain represents repressed anger turned more safely on the self than on boss, parent, or spouse. Maybe, but if back spasms are caused by emotion, how come they can be cured by exercise? A strong back can take the strain of stress.

The Anatomy of a Back

The vertebrae of the backbone are like beads through which the spinal cord is strung from the lower spine to where the cord enters the brain at the back of the skull. Between each vertebra and the next one is a cushion covered with cartilage and stuffed with gelatin — the disk that keeps the bones from rubbing against each other. Nerves branch out from the spinal cord through channels between vertebrae and reach from there to the arms, legs, hands, feet, toes, and fingers whose muscles they activate. Sensory nerves — the ones that bring you temperature and touch — run in the opposite direction, from the skin inward to the spinal cord.

In stiff-backed creatures like birds and horses, long-spurred vertebrae interlock, giving the backbone a degree of built-in rigidity. The vertebrae in our more bendable backs aren't self-supporting. What's more, the human backbone in its oddly upright position is subjected to vertical compression rather than bearing the pull of gravity along its length as it does in other animals. In addition, we carry a heavy head.

A textbook backbone, seen in profile, is shaped like a mildly

Back Facts

There are just a few things you ought to know. The lowest estimate for the proportion of Americans of all ages who will suffer back pain at some time in their lives is 50 percent; some estimates are as high as 80 percent. We spend, as individuals, $13 billion per year to relieve back pain. The economy loses too. Back pain is the leading cause of missed work after the common cold, and these absences cost an estimated $5 billion in lost earnings and productivity.

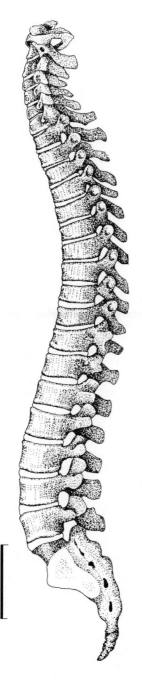

neck vertebrae

thoracic (chest) vertebrae
to which the ribs attach

lumbar, or lower back, vertebrae

sacrum to which
the hips attach

coccyx, or tailbone

The smooth, round portions of the vertebrae face inward, toward the belly; they are separated by disks. The protruding spines that jut to the rear are the bumps you can feel running along the middle of your back. Beyond the large vertebrae of the lower back is a fused section called the sacrum, which connects to the hip bones. The very bottom, also fused, is the coccyx, or tailbone.

curved *S*. The curve gives the back a little spring and distributes weight evenly all along the spine so that no one portion bears a greater burden than another. But the load is supposed to be shared by muscles. Think of a loin of pork or a standing rib roast: Those chops are ribs, attached to vertebrae, and if you've ever sliced a roast beef, you know that it is largely held together by its meat, the muscle of the beast. The muscles that run along your spine are the same meat. The thinner they are, the less strongly they buttress the backbone. Gravity presses the vertebrae against one another, squeezing the disks between them. The weight of head, chest, shoulders, and arms bends the upper back into too deep a curve, and the lower back is pulled too straight.

I mentioned ribs. Those on pork chops have been cut short; their front ends, which in life circle the pig's chest, are spareribs. The rib cage is, of course, part of the whole body support structure. So, however, are the abdominal muscles (bacon in a pig, flank steak in beef). Abdominal muscles attach to the backbone, the rib cage, the hips, and to one another. Ideally, your trunk really is a trunk, a firm cylinder all the way around that shares the weight evenly and does the work equably. When abdominal muscles can't hold their own, back muscles have to be in continual contraction to even keep you upright. That contraction sways the back into too deep a lower curve.

A weak belly or a weak back (or a weak trunk altogether) especially strains the muscles that run along the lower spine. They are always being pulled, they are always resisting, and they simply get exhausted with the effort. Simple exhaustion can throw a muscle into spasm, an abnormal contraction that feels like a knot, hurts like the devil, and won't let go for days.

Bending or lifting is often the last straw for already beleaguered muscles, and so is a twist, as in slapping a fly on your shoulder, or a jerk, as in grabbing for a falling glass of milk, or any awkward movement that catches the back off balance. Then muscle and tendon may tear.

An unnaturally curved back also strains the ligaments that strap vertebrae together. They can tear too. Any of these injuries also sends muscles into spasm.

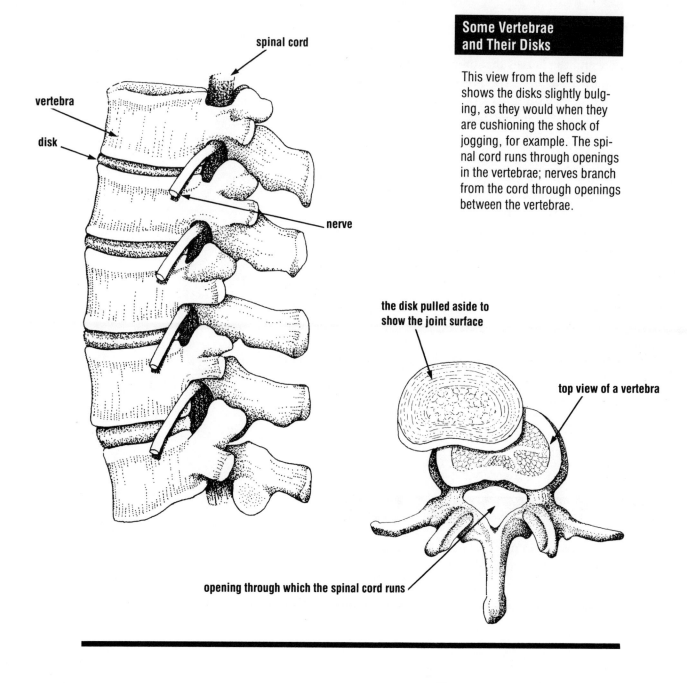

spinal cord

vertebra

disk

nerve

Some Vertebrae and Their Disks

This view from the left side shows the disks slightly bulging, as they would when they are cushioning the shock of jogging, for example. The spinal cord runs through openings in the vertebrae; nerves branch from the cord through openings between the vertebrae.

the disk pulled aside to show the joint surface

top view of a vertebra

opening through which the spinal cord runs

The pain caused by tears or muscle exhaustion is called simple backache. Complicated back pain is caused by damage to the disks between vertebrae and the nerves that branch out from the spine. Weak back muscles allow disks to be compressed too much or squished out to one side. The disk may rupture — not as in "splat"; it's more usually a break about the size of a pinhole that allows some of the disk's gelatinous filling to leak out. Neither a compressed disk nor a leaky one is plump enough to cushion the joint well; that in itself is painful. Worse, nerves in the vicinity are pinched, or squeezed, by extruded jelly. As you may know from a painful experience at the dentist's, nerves don't like being pinched and squeezed.

So check out your trunk. Go ahead; look at it in the mirror. If it doesn't remind you of a tree in any way, you'd best take this short strengthening course for back and belly. Another way to check your trunk strength is to imagine rolling a boulder uphill or rowing a boat against the wind. If you get tuckered out just thinking about it, your body's probably become at least dimly aware of its deficiencies and needs your help.

One warning, though: This strengthening course is for weak but otherwise healthy backs. Don't try the exercises without checking with your doctor if your back hurts now or if you've ever had an injury to a disk or nerve.

One Tightener, Two Lifts, and a Setter Dog

You can give yourself a solid trunk in about a month by doing the four exercises here every day. *Every day.* This is a crash course, not a maintenance program.

You already know the isometric belly tightener, although I'll repeat it for your convenience. The others are new.

Pull in your abdomen: Breathe normally while pulling in your tummy as far as it will go. Aim for your spine! Hold that tummy in until some distraction makes you forget what you were doing. As soon as you remember that you forgot, do the exercise again. The aim is to make a taut belly a habit, not an exercise.

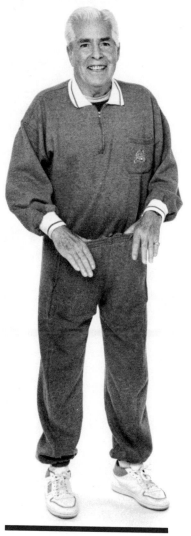

Lift your head and shoulders: This less demanding version of a sit-up strengthens the belly without bending the back.

Lie on the floor on your back, put your hands behind your head, and stare at a spot on the ceiling. Pretend you're holding a grapefruit under your chin; that will keep your head tilted slightly back. Now lift yourself so that your shoulder blades are off the ground. Hold the lift for a count of three, and work toward a total of ten lifts.

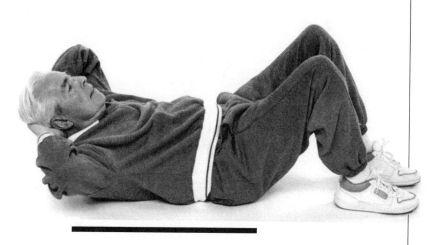

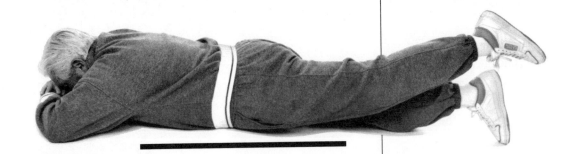

Lift your legs: Now turn over on your belly. Rest your head on your folded arms. Lift one leg up — a couple of inches is all that's necessary — hold it there for a count of three, and let it down again. Do the same with the other leg. Then lift both legs for a count of three. Repeat each of these lifts five times for a total of fifteen lifts.

Pose like a setter dog: This amusing exercise is for back muscle balance; it strengthens both sides of the back alternately but equally.

Get up on your hands and knees. Lift your left arm and right leg out straight, and hold them there for a count of three. Shift to the right arm and left leg, and hold them out for the same amount of time. Repeat ten times per side for a total of twenty.

Two clues will tell you that you're making progress with these exercises: when they become easier to do, and when it doesn't hurt at all to do them. If your muscles are really slack, you'll feel the strain of sucking in your gut in your lower back as well as in your belly. The other exercises may leave you somewhat sore at first. By the end of the month, your trunk will be considerably stronger, and the exercises will be a cinch.

What if they were a cinch in the first place? Well, maybe you didn't need them. At least not yet.

I'd recommend that everyone add the back and belly exercises to their regular thrice-weekly routine as insurance against unnoticed slackening. Backs often don't complain until that last straw hits.

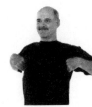

SIX

A Good Brisk Walk

*L*et's say you've done your stretch and strength exercises for six weeks now: Your legs and arms are stronger, your joints are noticeably more flexible. I hope you've also chosen to build a firm trunk. Are you now fit?

Not necessarily.

Although the word *fitness* is loosely used as a synonym for robust, its medical meaning is much narrower. Fitness is a measure of how much effort you can expend without getting out of breath. A person may be strong but not fit or weak but fit; suppleness doesn't enter the picture at all. Unfortunately, fitness has become so entangled in marathons and other heroics that you might not have known that huffing and puffing — or not huffing and puffing — have anything to do with it. Worse, you might have thought the road to fitness was too grueling to travel at your age. Not so. Not if you walk there.

I'm not sure you ought to get there any other way unless maybe through swimming, which is a great way to go, or some hobby like dog training, backpacking, or bird watching that requires trekking. Golf may seem like a good choice, but golfers tend to amble over the course at a pace that's better for their social life than for their physical fitness.

I have had patients who still sprinted in their seventies, but, mind you, they were patients. Although I appreciate the torn knees, twisted elbows, and other athletic injuries from which I mostly earn my living, I don't recommend banging your body to fitness. The irony of the bang-yourself-to-fitness craze that has consumed our generation is that the longer life we aim to get isn't going to be much fun to lead under a bowed back on hobbled knees.

The Minimum Walk

All you need to do to get fit and stay that way is walk briskly for half an hour to an hour a day. By brisk, I mean at a pace you would use when you really want to get somewhere, but not so fast that you feel uncomfortable. Since I don't know your age or condition, I can't tell you exact speeds in miles per hour. To me, a leisurely stroll is about two miles per hour; three miles per hour is a determined pace; four to five miles per hour is brisk. If you're eighty, your brisk might be my leisurely. If you're ninety, a half hour's walk might get you once around the block. We're not measuring miles here.

The pace ought to make you breathe more deeply and more rapidly than usual, but you should be able to carry on a conversation as you walk. In fact, I recommend that you find a walking companion. The time will be more pleasantly spent, you'll hardly notice that you're exercising, and you'll be helping a friend to fitness on the way.

Walking is an aerobic exercise: It steps up your need for oxygen. As your body uses more oxygen, your heart and lungs accommodate. You breathe faster to bring in more oxygen; your heart pumps blood faster and harder to pick up the extra supply of oxygen at the lungs and deliver it speedily to the rest of the body. These accommodations happen right away.

Other, more gradual accommodations are those that make you fit. Arteries, including those that supply the heart, grow wider and branch more. Fatty deposits that constrict those arteries diminish, and the proportion of "good," high-density cholesterol (HDL) increases at the expense of "bad," low-density cholesterol (LDL). These changes improve heart performance and possibly protect from heart attack.

Just as important, more blood gets to the muscles that move your body. They, too, are able to perform better — to work harder and longer without tiring. You'll notice that you can walk farther, and probably faster, within two weeks. Soon you'll notice a difference in your breathing: You'll be able, when you're aerobically fit, to climb hills without breathlessness. Your heart won't thump with the effort, either. Your muscles will get enough oxygen without your having to pant and pound for them.

From a Muscle's Point of View

All this takes some explaining. What is oxygen for? Why do muscles need it? What actually happens in your body as you walk?

All cells need oxygen for respiration, a chemical process in which the fuels you eat — fats, proteins, sugars, starches — are taken apart step by step, into very small molecules. At each step in the process, the energy that held the pieces of the food molecule together is

A Mitochondrion, Partly Dissected

The outer membrane of a mitochondrion encloses a second, very convoluted membrane, both shown here partly cut away to reveal the complex structure. Respiration is conducted by teams of highly specialized molecules, known only in bacteria and mitochondria, that dwell within and on the surfaces of the inner chamber.

released and is then available to build your body, to heat it, and to move it.

The process begins with fermentation, the way in which bacteria get energy: Food molecules are chopped into largish pieces, one of which is that villainous lactic acid that tuckers muscles out. But leftovers of fermentation are the necessary kindling for respiration. A muscle fiber that has sufficient oxygen burns up lactic acid as fast as it accumulates. All that's left after respiring a food molecule is carbon dioxide and water, plus thirty-two times more energy than fermentation alone provides.

Respiration doesn't happen out in the sloshy wetness of a cell. It goes on inside very complex, minute cell organs called mitochondria, which, believe it or not, were originally respiring prey swallowed (but not digested) by our one-celled ancestors. Mitochondria now live semi-autonomous lives inside our cells, using genes of their own to make the specialized chemicals needed for respiration and reproducing independently of the cell they inhabit. Although muscle fibers don't reproduce, their mitochondria do, and at a rate geared to the muscle's respiratory needs. Walking briskly creates a need that mitochondria then fill by multiplying. More mitochondria can then consume more leftovers and supply more energy for the muscle to continue moving harder and longer than it could before.

Naturally, though, more mitochondria need more oxygen. Panting is one way to provide extra oxygen, because the more frequently the lungs are filled, the more oxygen there is for the red blood cells to pick up and deliver. Deliveries can be speedier, too, because the heart pumps faster. The need to breathe hard and pump fast, however, signals the blood vessels to enlarge their capacity. Large ones widen; little ones branch. Soon the need to pant and thump subsides as rich networks of capillaries become able to satisfy the demands of oxygen-hungry muscles and their multiplying mitochondria even if you walk or work for hours at a time. Aerobic fitness comes about through microscopic changes, but you feel it in a big way.

Of course, the catch is that you have to make an effort to achieve effortlessness. The microscopic doings of blood vessels and cell organs is in response to the demands you place on them, and the only language they understand is the chemistry of your effort.

The Difference Between A Little and A Lot

The wonderful new news is that a smallish effort yields a surprisingly large return. The greatest health gain comes from getting off that couch and walking daily. Out of every thousand sedentary men, sixty-five can be expected to die this year. Were they all to take a walk instead of sitting down all day, forty fewer would die. Greater gains may come with greater fitness, but the differences in the death rate between people who walk a mile a day and people who run thirty miles a week is not dramatic and, I believe, not worth it.

Bonuses

I learned long ago not to buy new shoes in the morning. Feet are at their smallest then; by the middle of the afternoon, shoes that fit at ten will surely be too tight.

Swollen feet and ankles result from a less than impressive system for circulating fluids upstream to the heart, against the pull of gravity. Blood circulation is a loop: Blood is pumped from the heart through arteries to, say, your left foot, flows through a bed of capillaries there, and returns through veins to the heart. The pumping pressure drops to zero at the bottom of this run. How can the blood climb the uphill route back home?

Within all veins are simple one-way valves. Blood can flow through the valves going upstream but can't fall back again. Since by the time blood enters the veins it is beyond range of the heart's pumping power, the only force to push it upward is muscle squeeze, like a fist around a tube of toothpaste. Flexing a calf squeezes blood up the leg.

Blood isn't the only liquid in your legs, however. When plasma leaks from capillaries to deliver oxygen and nutrients to nearby cells, it joins the body fluid that bathes your innards everywhere. Some body fluid leaks back into the capillaries to thin the blood enough for its return trip. But a second circulatory system, the lymphatic system, also picks up body fluid to cleanse it of dead cells and other stray debris in the lymph nodes (like the ones you can feel nestled in your groin) before dumping it back into a large vein near the heart. Lymph vessels have the same simple one-way valves that veins have, and lymph fluid is similarly squeezed toward the heart by flexing muscles.

Just being upright all day swells the feet with some extra fluid; the excess drains back to the heart during the night. This normal situation worsens with sitting or standing jobs that require no walking. The

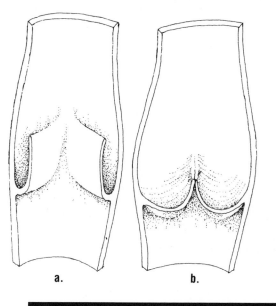

a.   b.

A Valve in a Vein

a. The pressure of contracting muscles against the vein forces blood up through the valve.
b. The valve then collapses shut, preventing blood from falling back down.

Varicose Veins

The valves in varicose veins don't close correctly; blood slips back down through them, distending the vein to twice or more its usual size. Varicose veins are common in the lower legs, where the blood flow is sluggish and the trip uphill is hard. Seriously swollen varicose veins sometimes require surgery, but even mildly swollen veins ache by the end of the day.

You can relieve this pain, and also reduce the swelling of the veins, by wearing elastic socks or stockings. The extra pressure against the veins helps to squeeze blood upward and restricts the space in which the blood can pool. At night, sleeping with your feet up on several pillows lets the pooled blood flow downhill from your legs.

In moderate cases, these two measures can return varicose veins almost to their normal size in a month or two.

---

muscles aren't flexed often enough. Blood accumulates in the veins, lymph accumulates in the lymph vessels, and, because the whole drainage system flows so sluggishly, body fluid, too, accumulates among the cells. Your feet and ankles become especially sodden; your hands swell too. The remedy, of course, is to swing your arms and stride along to keep your rivers running — in short, a walk.

By the way, a daily constitutional also keeps the brain's endorphins dripping. Think of a walk as a healthier version of the "happy hour."

How to Spare the Time

Perhaps you can walk to work or to the train station to meet the minimum goal of a half hour's outing daily with no more disruption to your schedule than arising a little earlier than usual. Or use your lunch hour. Eat at your desk while doing busywork, then take off for a walk. For high-powered Wall Street types who like to know exactly what they've gained for every hour spent, twenty city blocks equals about a mile, and a broker below retirement age may do eighty blocks — four miles — in a lunchtime.

Those who don't work or have retired can walk anytime, but that's a problem. When is it "natural" to take a walk when most of the day is free? Husband and wife might like to take an evening stroll together. Friends might set aside the time they often chat or visit to take a walk instead.

Naturally, walking *to* somewhere is more motivating than walking around in circles. That's easy for city folks; walking to get from here to there is often faster and less frustrating than being stalled in traffic, and a goal, such as a movie theater, department store, or friend's home, is often within walking distance. Suburbia doesn't oblige in the same way, but it certainly beats sidewalks and storefronts for natural beauty. And villages beat suburbia: Within walking distance of a friend's cottage in Maine are (1) the village, (2) a swimming hole, (3) the lobster pound (just caught and half the price stores charge), (4) gorgeous wildflowers, (5) fiddlehead ferns, chantarelle mushrooms, blackberries, raspberries, cranberries, crabapples, clams, and mussels for the picking, plucking, and digging, (6) sunset over the harbor viewed from Armbrust Hill. My friend walks; who wouldn't walk in paradise?

Some people in the suburbs have taken to walking in malls. A very old woman I know — she's well over ninety now — gets some of her walking done in the supermarket. Capable only of hobbling with a cane, she nevertheless sails along behind a shopping cart.

But she insists on lugging an enormous pocketbook, and I say shuck it.

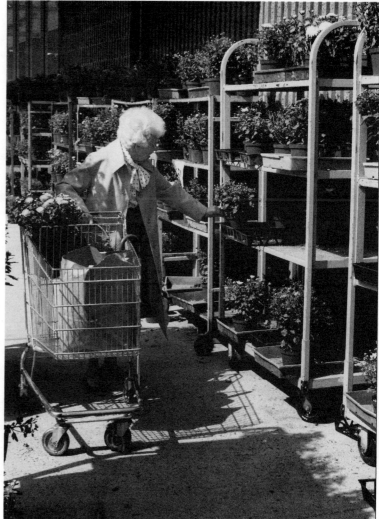

Ninety-four, and still going strong behind a shopping cart

To get the most out of a walk, and to enjoy it more, do whatever you can to free yourself of paraphernalia. You want your back straight, your head up, and your arms swinging freely.

Try to find an uncrowded route where you don't have to dodge other pedestrians, bicycles, baby carriages, and dogs. That's not so easy in a big city, and the other option — finding a deserted route — can be dangerous where muggings are common. But try. Residential areas are usually less congested than shopping streets; often a crosstown walk has fewer obstacles than along the main street. Parks may be perfect on weekdays and in winter, though not often on summer Sundays.

Speaking of the weather, don't let it keep you in. Walking in the rain can be very pleasant unless it's cold and driving. Waterproof yourself in rubber boots, a slicker, and a broad-brimmed rain hat that sheds water on your shoulders, not your face. Juggling an umbrella will only hamper your stride, and everyone else's.

Sure, it's dumb to walk abroad when the wind-chill factor makes the temperature equivalent to minus twenty, but a still, cold day shouldn't stop you if you dress properly. That means lined footwear or an extra pair of socks, layered clothing or winter woollies (which these days come in comfortable silk, my favorite), pants, not breezy skirts, and a coat with a snug, turn-up collar. I'd like to give clothing manufacturers a piece of my mind about women's coats. They're never warm enough or wide enough or light enough for winter walking comfort. A down jacket may be better. A warm hat is a must. And I insist that patients who come to me in the winter bundle their neck in a cozy scarf; whatever I can do to relax their muscles is undone the moment they hunch themselves again against the cold.

In summer's sultry weather, walk in the morning or evening, not in the high heat of noon.

As you get used to walking as a means of transportation, you may find you need to revise your wardrobe, especially if you're a woman. A woman simply can't walk normally in high or even medium heels — or, in fact, in most shoes created for the sake of looks instead of locomotion. High heels shorten the calf muscles and shorten the step, not to mention strain the back. Then there's the big toe, which, when not scrunched, supports the arch and is the major springboard for each forward launch. Men, you read this too, because plenty of classy men's shoes are also too pointy-toed for easy walking.

Take off your shoes. Notice your foot. The fatty pads of the heel and ball are level, unlike in a shoe, in which the heel is raised. Take a step in slow motion. Watch and feel what's happening. Your heel touches the ground first, and, as your weight shifts forward, your foot rolls until your weight is on the ball of it. Then, as you continue the forward roll, your toes — especially that big toe — dig in, pushing you forward. Quickly, before you lift that foot, look at your toes. They are somewhat splayed, giving you a broad as well as a muscular launching pad. Or they should be if your pointed shoes haven't permanently bent

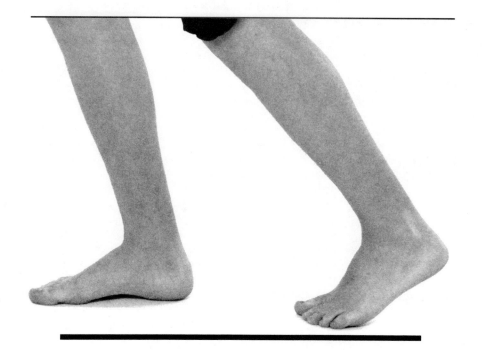

them inward. That pushing action of the toes also supports your arch — you can actually feel the tension there — in a way that's not possible when they're scrunched together. Long walks in tight shoes press your toes, bend them, and leave your arches aching.

A good walking shoe should be something like an outer foot. It shouldn't require any more effort to hold it on than it does to hold your skin in place when you walk. That means it should hug your heel and embrace your arch firmly. The sole should be padded and springy, like your own sole. You ought to be able to wiggle your toes in it.

If you're making a round trip to and from home, you can wear these shoes without having to carry the snazzier shoes you're going to wear after the walk. Since you don't need to powder your nose while walking, you don't need a pocketbook, either. Wear something with a pocket and stash your wallet there. If you're on the way to work, you'll probably have to carry the high heels or the tasseled loafers, and that will burden one arm. Nothing cramps one's walking style like the clutch of a purse or the drag of a gym bag or briefcase. A backpack would solve the problem, but I know a lot of readers over fifty won't like that idea much.

I try.

Needless to say — but I'm saying it anyway — tight pants and narrow skirts are no good for walking.

The Ideal Stride

Tight muscles and joints aren't good for walking, either. Sometimes it's been so long since a person has moved freely that his gait has shortened to accommodate the tightness. You mustn't let your walking gait diminish into what will eventually become a totter. Sneak a look at yourself in windows as you walk by to see if you can catch a glimpse of your walking style. Does your chin stick out? Are your shoulders hunched? Are your arms clutched or stuck into your pockets? All these reflect poor walking style. Rate the length of your gait against that

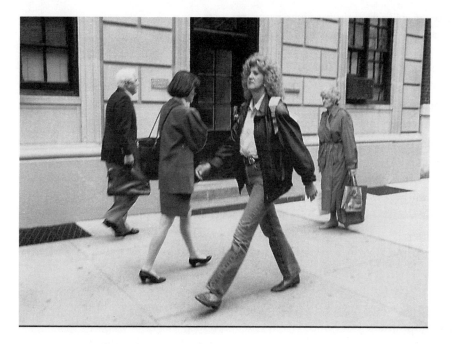

of your walking companions. Unless you have unusually short legs or are already in your eighties, you shouldn't always have to hasten to keep up.

If you don't pass these tests, there could be two things wrong. First, you might be crunched from anxiety even though you are actually limber enough to walk tall and stride smartly. I'm not a psychiatrist, but I have a homespun theory that seems to work. It's something like the song "I Whistle a Happy Tune" from *The King and I.* If you make yourself stride along as though you hadn't a care in the world, the worldly cares that weigh you down will lighten as you walk. It works for me; there's no harm in trying.

The other possibility is that your muscles and sinews are too stiff to express your carefree mood. Work on those stretches! And make your walks into stretching exercises too by purposely taking longer strides, swinging your arms in long arcs, and trying always to hold your head taller than the pedestrians around you. As you can imagine, the fewer steps per mile, the less tiring the walk.

Finally, walking will be like dancing — rhythmic, refreshing, fun to do. Which reminds me: Marching songs were written to aid in walking, and humming a Sousa tune as you march along will keep you stepping smartly. I'm also reminded that dancing is excellent aerobic exercise for those over fifty, provided the style doesn't require leaping or swinging your partner through the air. I'd vote for ballroom or country dancing. The latter is undergoing a revival noted for its acceptance, indeed enthusiasm, among people of every age.

Another alternative is swimming. In fact, swimming is in some ways superior to walking or dancing. You float: There's no gravity to contend with and therefore no impact to your knees or hips, no flattening of your arch, no pressure on your spine. Yet water resists your movements through it, so your muscles must work harder than when walking through air. And more muscles are used. Walking does little for weak abdominals, but notice when you swim how your belly tenses as you kick your legs. Because you're "on all fours" in the water — pushing with all your limbs — your arms, shoulders, and back are worked. Those muscles aren't used much in walking. Swimmers are noticeable among athletes for the smooth, even way in which their muscles develop. Bicyclists, by comparison, become thick in the legs, but their arms and tummies are nothing to write home about. The classic crawl is also a natural stretching exercise: A swimmer's muscles are long, not bulgy like a weight lifter's.

Of course, it's hard for many people to find a place to swim on a regular basis, especially for free. For money, there are town and club pools in the suburbs, and swimming is always possible in the city for a fee. A friend of mine made arrangements to swim for nothing in a neighbor's pool on weekdays while the neighbor is at work, summers only. Who has a friend with a heated pool?

That's another nice thing about walking. It's so egalitarian.

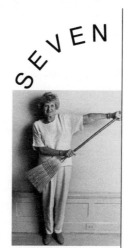

SEVEN

Hints for the Hurt

Foraging through fitness news at the New York Academy of Medicine's library, I reaped a bumper crop of discouraging statistics. Some twenty million sports injuries are reported every year. Even among golfers, 65 percent suffer injuries of one sort or another from playing their game. Half the population — some estimates are as high as 80 percent — suffer back pain at some time in their lives. A quarter of the population of women over fifty have osteoporosis. Arthritis is almost guaranteed to strike everyone who lives to four score years and ten.

Not that I don't see, eight hours a day, five days a week, a parade of injured bodies, but I had thought my view of a population bent with pain was biased by my profession. Now I realize that there must be lots of you out there who hurt, and quite a few of you who hurt so much that at the moment you can't do the exercises I suggest.

Can't or shouldn't. Not without your doctor's say-so. Exercises helpful for strained backs may hinder the healing of injured disks. Isometrics are good for maintaining muscle strength while a broken bone is healing, but they put a surprisingly heavy strain on the heart, and cardiac patients are advised to shun them. I say again, as I've said before, only your doctor knows for sure what's safe for you.

With that warning fresh in your mind, I think I can safely cover a few common ailments and suggest what kinds of physical therapy a doctor, encouraged by a patient's eagerness to do *something*, might prescribe.

My first, and most important, suggestion is to call your doctor when you first feel pain. Pain wasn't invented to test your fortitude. It evolved in animals as primitive as octopuses, which presumably have no moral character to test. Pain is a warning that something is damaged, and even an octopus knows to pull a tentacle away from a pinch.

Unfortunately, pain indicates only the general location of the damage, not what has caused it, not what to do about it, and sometimes not even how serious it is. So your knee hurts. Take a look at the picture of a knee joint on page 92 and tell me whether you hurt in a miniscus or a bursa. There are several dozen possible injuries to a knee, and pain can't say which one you've got. That's a doctor's job.

Any injury, even a scratch that doesn't break the skin, causes inflammation. Scratch the inside of your arm and watch the scratch line redden and puff up. A more damaging wound would soon become hot and painful. Inflammation — redness, swelling, heat, and pain — is a chemical event of astonishing complexity that involves not only substances released by damaged cells but, upon that chemical signal, many other kinds of mobile cells that gather at the site to exercise damage control and encourage healing.

One group of chemicals, called prostaglandins, stimulate pain nerve endings. That first alert is meant to tell you to protect the injured area. Prostaglandins also signal certain cells to secrete histamine, which dilates blood capillaries in the neighborhood and makes them leakier than usual. More blood flows to the area — that's the redness you see and the extra heat you feel. The extra heat, as well as the extra oxygen and nutrients in the greater supply of blood, speeds up the activities of healthy cells so that they can divide more often and make more of the products necessary to healing. An extra quantity of clear blood plasma leaks from the capillaries — that's the swelling — and white blood cells, the body's cleanup crew, slither out too. They eat germs if any are around and also scavenge for dead body cells and broken fibers. The chemical goings-on also attracts fibroblasts, which set to work repairing torn fibers.

Inflammation is therefore not the damage itself but a necessary prelude to healing. However, too much inflammation for too long can hurt healthy tissue, and the cells that emit these fiery chemicals aren't awfully good at deciding when enough's enough.

That's why the first thing a doctor is likely to prescribe even before your injury can be diagnosed is ice, aspirin, and rest: a trio of therapies that reduce inflammation.

Cooling the injured area with ice shrinks the capillaries and slows cell activity, including that of pain neurons and inflammatory chemical secreters. You hurt less, and the swelling goes down. Aspirin or aspirin substitutes such as ibuprofen and acetaminophen inhibit the production of prostaglandins and so also relieve the pain and swelling. Resting the injured part — by putting an arm in a sling, a leg on a chair, a back on a bed — avoids any further damage that might call up more troops.

By rest I mean no more than twenty-four hours before, by getting to a doctor, you find out whether resting any longer is in order. Usually, it's not.

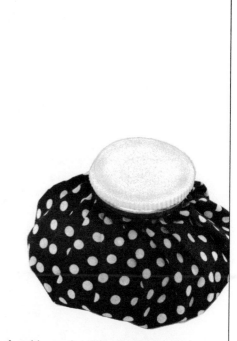

Ice Ideas

Although cooling an injury with ice cubes wrapped in a towel is a quick way to reduce swelling, it's a lumpy, cumbersome contraption to wrap around an elbow or an ankle. Crushed ice makes a snugger cold pack. Crush ice cubes in a towel by smashing them with the side of a hammer. Then arrange the crushed ice on another towel and fold it to the size and shape you need.

Another idea is to use one of those flexible plastic ice packs designed for picnic coolers. Let it thaw until it gets comfortably mushy. A family-size pack of frozen peas, slammed against the counter to separate them, has the consistency of a bean bag and is useful for cooling round joints like shoulders. You can also make your own cold pads with moistened cloth or paper towels folded to fit inside a plastic food storage bag and cooled in the freezer until cold but not stiff.

Then there's that standby, the ice bag that looks like a squashed hat; it was once popular for hangovers and is still sold at drugstores. Nothing has ever replaced it for comfort, convenience, and a willingness to stay where it is put.

RICE

RICE is the acronym doctors use to describe the standard treatment for ankle injuries, such as strains (when a muscle is injured by overuse) and sprains (when there is injury to ligaments or tendons as well). The initials stand for Rest, Ice, Compression, and Elevation. Rest means to keep your weight off the joint as much as possible, using a crutch or cane for support when walking is necessary. Ice means applying an ice bag or crushed ice wrapped in a small towel to reduce the pain and swelling. Compression is accomplished by wrapping the ankle in an elastic bandage, such as the Ace bandages sold by pharmacies. The bandage limits movement while the cells do their repair work. Elevation does *not* mean propping the foot on a stool or simply lying down. An injured ankle swells with body fluids. To keep the ankle drained, you must keep that foot above the level of your heart. That means propping it up on at least two plump and firm bed pillows — more if they are soft — and lying in that position for an hour at a time as many times a day as your doctor recommends and all night.

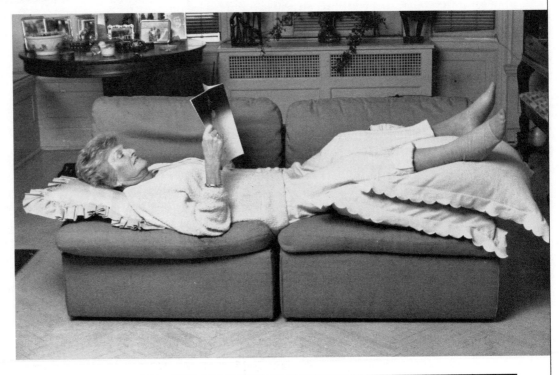

Resting can be hazardous. If you've strained your back, more than a day or two in bed will only weaken your muscles and make you more liable to reinjury when you at last arise. Recovery is not hastened; simple back pain (not involving damage to nerves or disks) goes away in one or two weeks with or without bed rest. Injured joints are particularly vulnerable to ill effects from long vacations: Fibers in an immobilized joint attach the joint surfaces to one another, preventing any motion at all. If you then try to move, you'll cry with pain. Believe me. On the other hand, going back to lifting crates or acing opponents on the tennis court with a bum back or a bad elbow isn't smart, either. What degree of activity may the doctor prescribe?

Sports medicine professionals have come up with the oxymoronic term "active rest" to describe a balance between the overuse that has usually caused the injury and the underuse that is likely to make it even worse. Active rest for a knee hurt by jogging might be walking or swimming. Active rest for a shoulder injured by serving might be playing doubles instead of singles or just hitting the ball for practice instead of playing an actual game. Active rest for a strained back usually involves going back to work, assuming that the job is less punishing than piano moving.

Strength and flexibility are inevitably lost during the acute stage of an injury, when you hurt too much to move. Weakness and rigidity most likely contributed to getting injured in the first place and will most likely do the same thing again. So full recovery requires specific exercises to strengthen your supporting muscles and to improve your range of motion. Aerobic exercise may be suggested to improve circulation, decrease pain, relax tension, and generally cheer you up. Posture is often an issue, especially with neck or back pain.

Necks

The neck stretches and isometric neck strengtheners in Chapter 3 are among those doctors are likely to prescribe for stiff and arthritic necks and even for whiplash injuries. I won't repeat them here.

Shoulders

The ball-and-socket joint of the shoulder is engineered to swing in a full circle and to swivel too. Such freedom of movement demands an elaborate arrangement of muscles, tendons, ligaments, and other structures, all of which are subject to injury and inflammation. The suffix "itis" denotes inflammation. These are some of the more common exercises your doctor might suggest for bursitis, tendonitis, arthritis, and other shoulder inflammations too numerous to name.

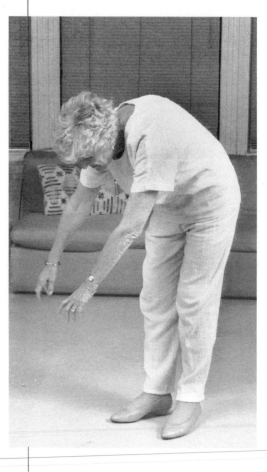

Codman's exercise: Dr. Ernest A. Codman, a Boston surgeon, devised this passive exercise to prevent frozen shoulder, in which fibers attach the joint surfaces to one another. The gentle swinging motion causes little pain, yet maintains enough mobility to keep fibers from locking the joint. The weight of the swinging arms also takes pressure off the joint and relaxes tense shoulder muscles.

Stand up, lean over, bend your knees slightly, and let both arms hang limp. Now move the upper part of your body around and around and back and forth, letting your arms swing as though they were vaguely stirring something. Don't use your shoulder muscles at all. Your arms should swing free like pendulums. Repeat the exercise often during the day for a few minutes at a time.

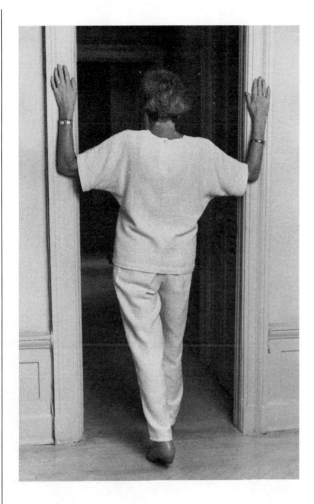

Doorway stretch: This stretches the front part of both shoulders. Stand in a doorway, put your forearms on the door frame with your hands at the level of your face, and take a step forward. If you can't feel the stretch try it again with a slightly longer step. Count to three, relax, and repeat ten times.

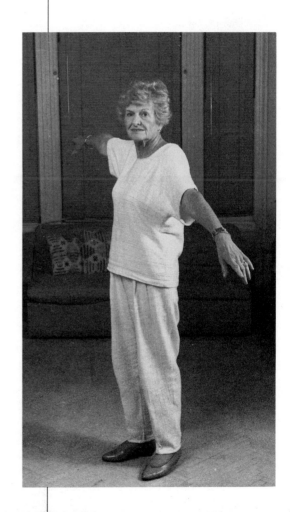

Sideways arm lift: To stretch the underside of the shoulder joint, stand up and lift both arms sideways until your hands are level with your shoulders — or, if you can't lift that far, as far as the injured arm will go before hurting. Hold the position for a count of three, relax, and repeat ten times.

Elbow pull: The elbow pull in Chapter 3 stretches the rear of the shoulder joint. Cock the injured arm in front of you, and with the other arm gently pull it across your chest. Same count, same repeat.

Elbows

Elbow joints are usually damaged by twisting motions. Tennis players tend to tear tissues at the outside of the elbow by twisting their forearm to the inside, as in a backhand stroke. Golfers damage the inside of the elbow by twisting outward during the follow-through of a swing. The fault may be in the player's form (get a pro to watch and correct your swing), but elbow injury is commonly caused by weak muscles in the forearm.

The exercises that follow may be prescribed to strengthen the forearm once healing is under way.

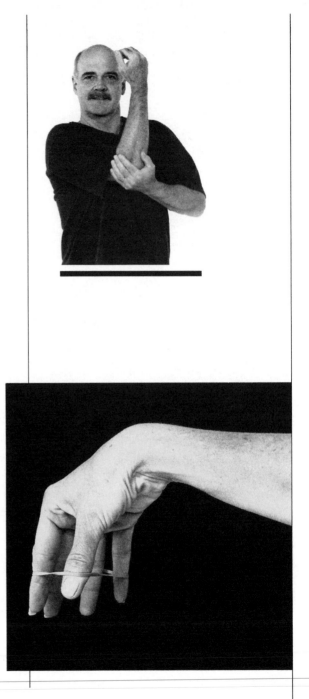

Rubber band stretch: Hold the injured arm out straight and support it at the elbow on the padded arm of a chair or sofa. Put a rubber band around your fingers and let the hand hang down. Work your forearm muscles by opening and closing your fingers against the pressure of the rubber band.

Weighted hand lift: This exercise can be done in the same position, on a couch or armchair, but using a dumbbell (or a can of soup). Hold the

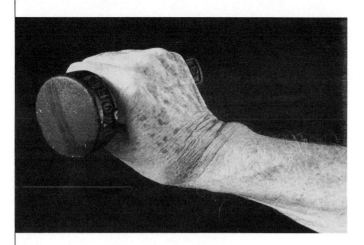
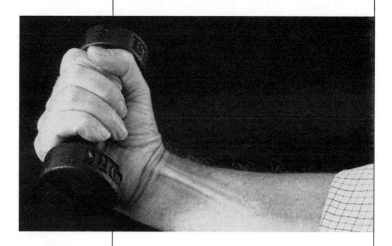

dumbbell in your hand with the palm facing down and lift your weighted hand ten times. Then turn your hand so that the palm is facing up and lift the dumbbell ten times again.

Backs

Your doctor may advise stretches for simple back pain after the acute stage of a back attack is over. Examples are the hip roll, knee pull, and leg straighten in Chapter 4. You may also be advised to begin a back and belly strengthening regime like the one in Chapter 5. Any treatment for nerve or disk damage would depend on what x-rays and other tests reveal.

The suggestions here are for people who have pulled ligaments or muscles in the lower back. They will keep the person reasonably active without throwing the back again into spasm while it is healing. The principle is to keep the back slightly swayed: not as swayed as that of a toddler showing off her belly button, but enough so that spinal ligaments aren't pulled taut and the ridges of muscle to both sides of the backbone aren't stretched.

To sleep: Sleep supine with a folded towel under the small of your back and a single pillow under your head. To get out of bed, roll onto your side, bring your knees up, and drop your feet over the side of the bed while using your arms to hoist yourself into a sitting position.

Reading or watching television while reclining bends your back the wrong way. Don't do it.

To bathe: Reclining in the bathtub also bends the back the wrong way. Take a shower.

To sit: Sit in a straight chair with a pillow at the small of your back. To get out of a chair without bending forward, wriggle to the front of the chair, then use your arms to push yourself to a standing position. To get into a car, back your behind into the seat using the door and doorframe for support. Then swing your legs in. Get out the opposite way, legs first.

TENS

TENS stands for Transcutaneous Electrical Nerve Stimulation, a therapy intended to relieve pain by "distracting" the pain nerve endings with pulses of low-level electricity delivered through the skin. The device, worn on a belt around the body, costs about $500, and over the last several decades it has been used by countless sufferers of chronic lower back pain.

The total amount spent by the American public for TENS has never been counted, but in 1986, the latest year for which figures are available, the U.S. Veterans Administration alone spent $2 million on the devices. Is this an endorsement?

Unfortunately, no. A recent study has shown that the Veterans Administration, as well as the gullible public, has thrown away its money. TENS does nothing to relieve chronic pain, or to reduce the number of episodes of acute pain, in those suffering from backache.

The study further showed just what you didn't want to hear: There is no easy solution. Exercise is the best cure for nagging back pain, and only strengthening your back and abdominal muscles makes episodes of acute back pain both less frequent and less severe.

To lift: To lift anything as heavy as groceries or a child, stand close, bend your knees, and let your legs do the work.

To stoop: To stoop as for vacuuming, flex your knees so that you can still keep your back arched.

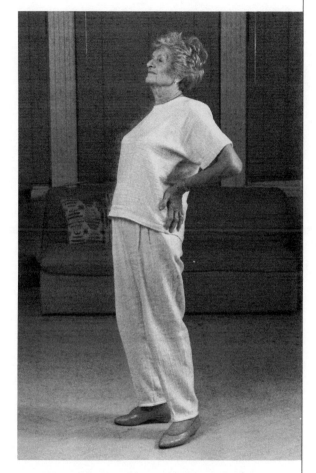

To stand: If you must stand for long periods of time, put your hands on your hips every few minutes, arch your back several times, and walk around a bit to relax the muscles.

To cough and sneeze: The normal chin-tucked, shoulder-hunched, back-bent way to cough or sneeze can send a sore back into spasm. Stand up, bend your knees, and arch your back before you let the cough or sneeze explode.

I've included these drawings of a knee, your body's biggest joint, to give you an idea of how complicated it is. Don't bother memorizing its many parts; just consider that any part can be injured. Twists, as in

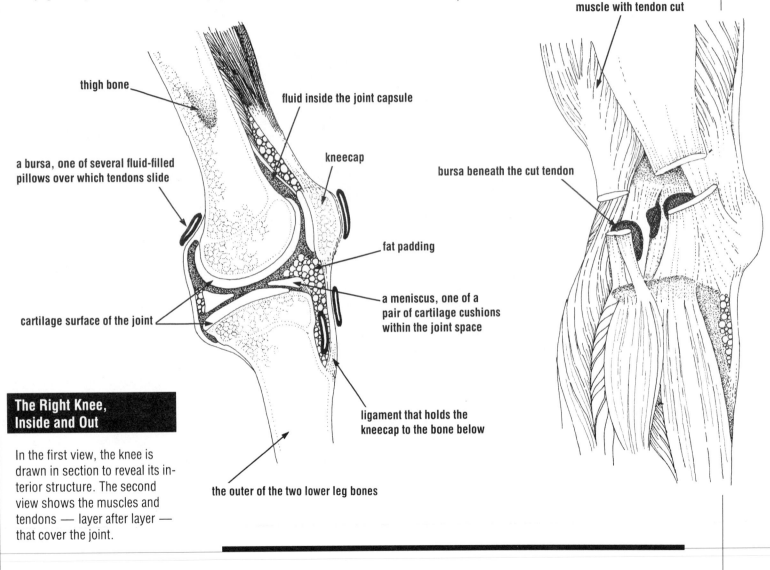

thigh bone

fluid inside the joint capsule

kneecap

muscle with tendon cut

a bursa, one of several fluid-filled pillows over which tendons slide

bursa beneath the cut tendon

fat padding

a meniscus, one of a pair of cartilage cushions within the joint space

cartilage surface of the joint

ligament that holds the kneecap to the bone below

the outer of the two lower leg bones

The Right Knee, Inside and Out

In the first view, the knee is drawn in section to reveal its interior structure. The second view shows the muscles and tendons — layer after layer — that cover the joint.

skiing, can tear ligaments and break cartilage. Pressure, as in kneeling, can inflame bursae. Pounding, as in running, can roughen the inner surface of the kneecap. Whatever the injury, the leg muscles that span the knee joint weaken very quickly while the person is limping toward recovery, and without strong muscles to support it, the knee is vulnerable to repeated injury in the future.

There are various "advanced," rather strenuous knee exercises that a doctor may prescribe for a knee injury once the pain has subsided enough to make them possible. Gentle exercises like the ones I describe here can be started right away.

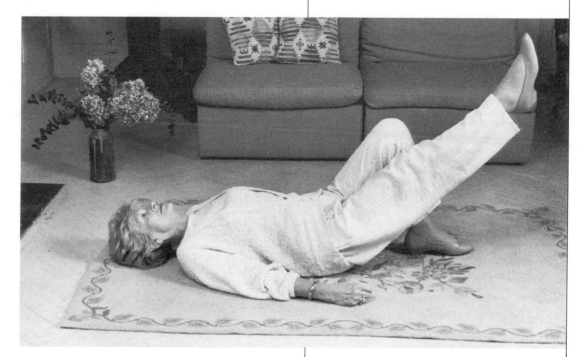

Leg lift: These leg lifts are the same as the weighted leg lifts described in Chapter 4, but without the weights. Lie on your back with the hurt leg straight and the other leg bent. Keep the hurt leg stiff, and lift it until both knees are level. Hold it for three seconds, then let it down. Repeat the lift ten times.

Thigh tighteners: These two isometrics will maintain strength in the big muscle at the front of the thigh and the hamstring muscle at the rear of the thigh. Lying with your injured leg straight and the other bent, stiffen the injured leg and try to push the back of the knee against the floor. That tightens the front of the thigh.

Now tighten the back of the thigh by pushing your heel into the floor. These exercises are usually done ten times apiece, holding the tightness each time for a count of three.

Knee cap bounce: Here's a casual toner you can do many times during the day while standing or sitting with the injured leg held straight. Just stiffen the leg, then relax it. The kneecap should bounce up when you tense, down when you relax.

Shins and Ankles

Shin splints — sharp pains in the muscles at the outside surface of the shin — are a symptom of muscle strain usually caused by too much walking or running on hard surfaces or in shoes that don't cushion well enough. The pain especially strikes people whose lower leg muscles aren't particularly strong. Because the lower leg muscles span and support the ankle joint, any weakness there also invites twisting injuries of the ankle.

These exercises to strengthen the lower leg are helpful therapy for shin splints and are also often prescribed to maintain or increase muscle strength after ankle and heel injuries.

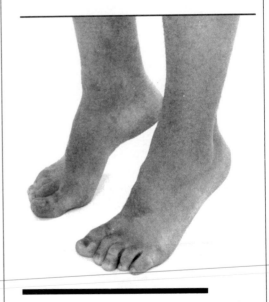

Tiptoes: This is an easy exercise. Stand up and raise yourself on tiptoe, then let yourself down again. There's no prescribed number of times. Let your muscles tell you when they're tired.

Weighted foot lifts and twirls: Instead of putting your ankle weights on your ankles, wrap one around the instep of each foot. Perch on the edge of a table so that your feet are off the floor. Bend each foot upward to lift the weight. Aim for fifteen lifts per foot, but settle for fewer at first if the exercise threatens to cramp your shin muscles.

When you're done lifting, twirl each weighted foot slowly, in a circle, as though you were writing the letter *O*. Again, your goal may be fifteen circles per foot, but stop short of that if your muscles are aching to quit.

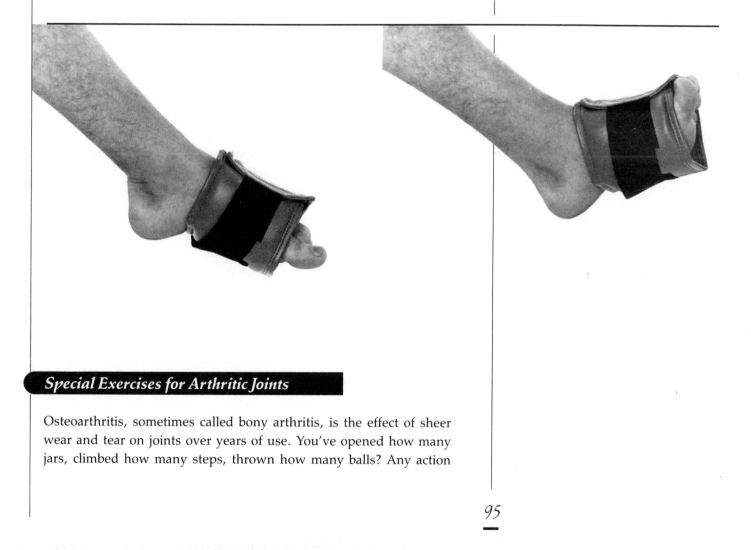

Special Exercises for Arthritic Joints

Osteoarthritis, sometimes called bony arthritis, is the effect of sheer wear and tear on joints over years of use. You've opened how many jars, climbed how many steps, thrown how many balls? Any action that repeatedly punishes cartilage joint surfaces gradually roughens and thins them like worn linoleum. A certain amount of damage is inevitable and irreparable.

Rheumatoid arthritis has a different cause and is much more severe. It is caused by autoimmunity, in which the body's own white blood cells, members of the immune community whose job is to destroy invading germs, attacks joint tissues as though they were the enemy. During an attack, the joint swells and reddens and may be excruciatingly painful. This inflammation does even more to damage the joint than the attack itself. The mainstay therapy for rheumatoid arthritis is therefore to suppress the inflammation with anti-inflammatory drugs and to forestall a further attack by dosing the immune cells with drugs that calm their ferocity.

Inflammation causes joint damage in osteoarthritis too. The knobby knuckles and stiff, sore joints of many older people are signs of inflammatory damage from osteoarthritis. To those disabilities, rheumatoid arthritis adds cruel, twisting joint distortion.

I'll describe here only a few common exercises that doctors are likely to prescribe. They are designed to keep wrists and fingers strong enough and straight enough to open car doors, unscrew jar tops, button buttons; shoulders limber enough to comb hair or reach for a can on a high shelf; hips, knees, and ankles free enough to walk upon.

None of the exercises should be done during a flare-up of inflammation, when rest is the right therapy and exercise is too painful, anyway. All are easier to do when the muscles are warm, as after a long, hot shower. None should be done beyond the point of pain — just until the movement hurts. And, unlike other exercises that are usually done once a day a few times a week, only exercising several times a day, seven days a week, will rebuild wasted muscles, increase the range of motion, and restore useful function to the damaged joints that may otherwise make arthritis sufferers unable even to fry an egg.

Homemade Hot Pads

Thank a friend's great-grandmother for this very modern hint. To make a reusable hot pad, moisten a terrycloth washcloth or hand towel and fold it into quarters. Place it inside a thin plastic bag, the kind that comes free on rolls in the supermarket (thicker plastic will get too hot to touch). Heat the bag in a microwave oven on high setting for 20 seconds. It will stay nice and hot for about 5 minutes and can be reheated as many times as needed. Thicker and softer microwavable hot pads are available in various sizes and shapes from pharmacies.

Arm circle: This exercise is for shoulder strength and flexibility. Standing, or sitting on a kitchen chair, let your arms hang straight by your sides. Lift the straightened arms as high as you can over your head. Then swing them back down to your sides. Stretch your arms during the entire swing up and down again as though you were inscribing in the air the largest possible circle your fingertips can reach.

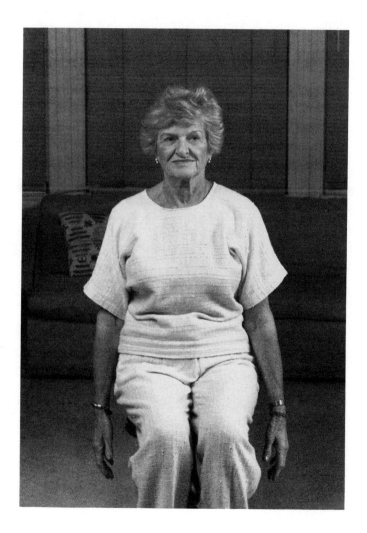

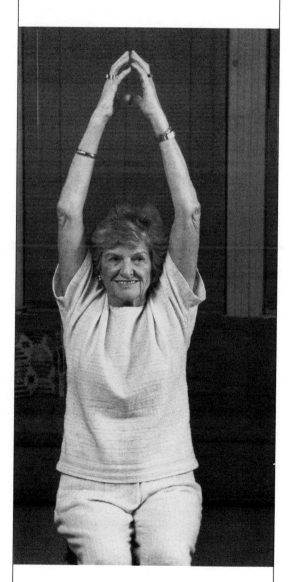

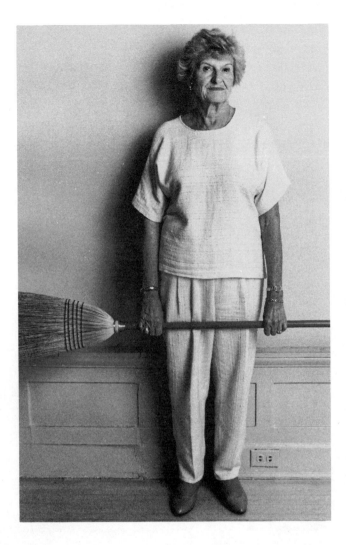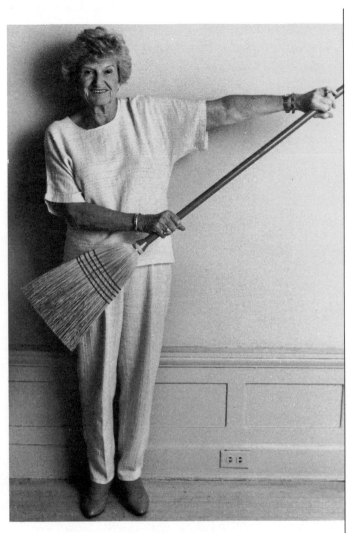

Stick lifts and swings: Broom, cane, yardstick, or dowel — it doesn't matter what kind of stick you use, just so it's long enough for you to grasp with your hands 2 to 3 feet apart, depending on your size.

Stand against a wall with your head, shoulders, heels, and behind touching it. Hold the stick in both hands and, with your elbows straight, lift it as high over your head as you can.

Still pressed to the wall, swing the stick from side to side. When you swing to the left, your right hand does the pushing and that elbow is bent. When you swing to the right, your left elbow bends to push the stick. The opposite arm, whose shoulder is being stretched by this exercise, is always straight.

Wrist twist: This exercise is designed to increase elbow rotation and strengthen the forearm muscles responsible for wrist power. You'll need a medium-weight hammer.

Grasp the hammer near its head. Hold your arm by your side with the elbow bent, as in serving a plate to someone. Turn your wrist from left to right, letting the weight of the hammer twist it farther than you are able to do alone; then turn the hammer back from right to left. Repeat the twist in both directions three or more times for each hand. As your range of motion improves, grip the hammer farther down the handle so that its weight works your muscles harder.

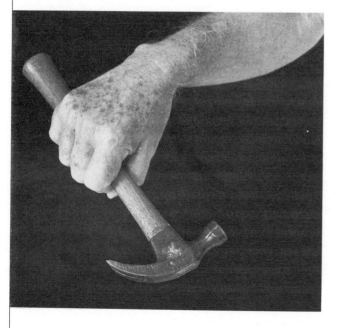

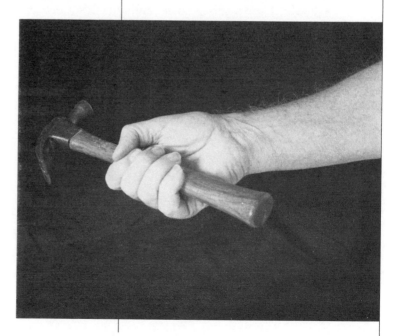

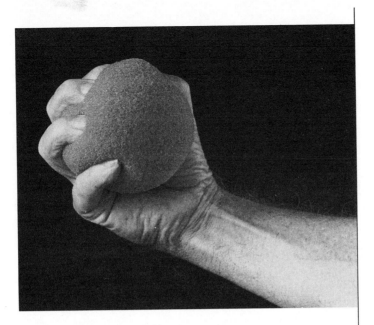

Hand squeeze: Keep a sponge ball handy for this exercise. Squeeze it repeatedly, alternating hands. Squeeze on the subway; squeeze during the news; squeeze while you're reading. Just think of yourself as Captain Queeg with an equally eccentric nervous habit.

Another prop for squeezing exercises is Silly Putty, which is somewhat more amusing to squeeze than a sponge ball and also requires more muscle. Use two or three globs of the stuff, enough to fill your fist.

Finger and wrist lifts: The point of this exercise is to strengthen the muscles that work your fingers and wrist; they are the only force you have to counteract twisting deformity in the many joints of the hands. The exercise also stretches hand ligaments that, when they are shortened with disuse, pull the hand into a claw.

Lay your hand flat on a table, the arm of a chair, or next to you in bed. If you can't get your palm flat, do the exercise anyway.

Spread your fingers as far as you can. Lift your index finger; then lift all the fingers (thumb included) together with your palm still pressed flat.

Then, to stretch your wrist and use a different set of muscles, lift your whole hand, keeping your forearm on the table, chair arm, or bed and flexing the wrist as far as possible.

These lifts should be done often during the day, whenever you're in a position to do them.

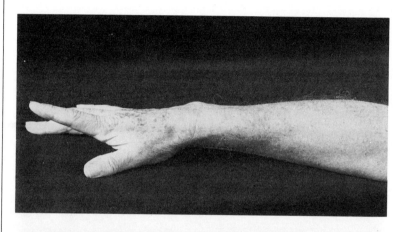

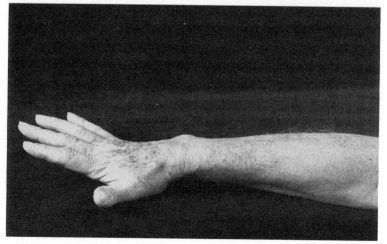

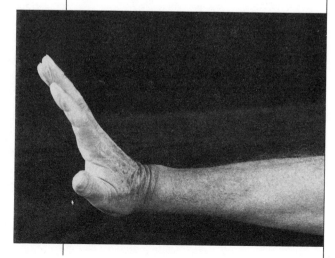

Chest expander: Ribs are jointed at the backbone, and arthritis can make those joints rigid. When your ribs don't move freely, the muscles in the chest wall weaken and breathing is restricted. This is a breathing exercise to improve the strength and flexibility of the chest and to keep the lungs able to expand to their full capacity.

When you're flat on your back in bed, inhale deeply while holding your hands against the sides of your rib cage. You should be able to feel your ribs pressing outward against your hands. Hold your breath for a second or two, then exhale. Repeating this a dozen times when you wake up, a dozen times when you go to bed, and, if you take a nap (I recommend it), a dozen more times in the afternoon should help to keep you breathing freely.

Hip stretcher: Lie on your back on the floor or in bed and point your toes together. Move one leg out to the side as far as it will go, then return it and move the other leg out to the side. This sideways stretch works well only if you keep your feet pigeon-toed.

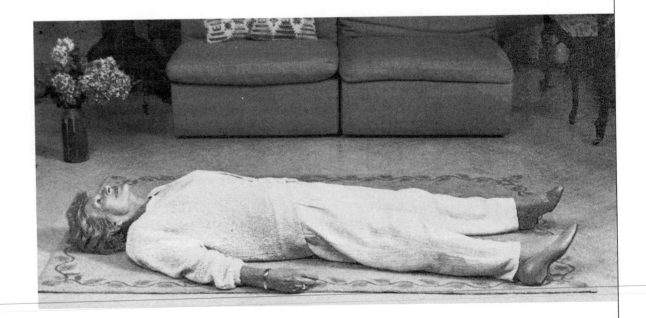

Knee pull: This is the same as the knee pull in Chapter 4. Lie on your back with your knees bent. Clasp your hands behind one knee and pull it back against your chest. The goal is to bend both the knee and the hip as far as they'll go, using the strength of your arms to coax the stiff joints. Repeat a few times for each leg several times a day.

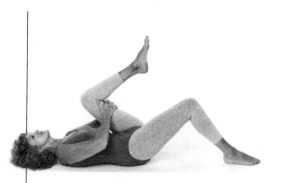

Heel lift: This exercise to straighten your knees and tighten the thigh muscles that support them can be done lying flat on the floor, in bed, or stretched out on a sofa. It's particularly helpful for people whose pain prevents them from walking to maintain strength and flexibility. Aim for a dozen heel lifts per day, divided among several sessions.

Push your thighs down to straighten your knees. If your knees won't straighten, put a rolled towel or small pillow under them and push your knees into it. Then lift your heels. The instructions usually say to lift an inch, but never mind the distance — it's the lifting effort, not the distance, that counts.

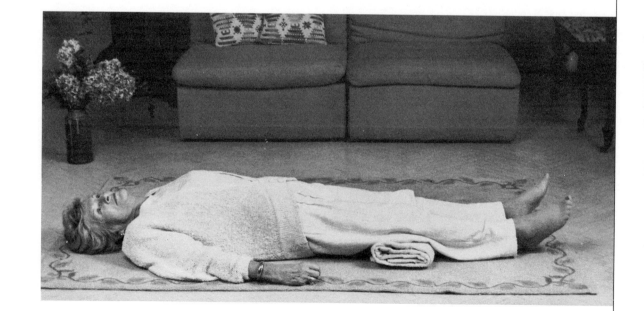

There was, in Victorian times, a category of people called invalids. A famous case was the poet Elizabeth Barrett, who, until enticed from her chaise longue by the robust Robert Browning, spent years exercising nothing but her strong and supple mind. You perhaps remember Colin in *The Secret Garden*, another invalid who was enticed back to health by Mary. Love can do wonders.

But what caused this once-common malady? It was an exaggerated belief in the need for rest in order to convalesce from an illness. Bed rest, let me remind you, is a wasting disease. If just weeks in bed can cost a person years of aging, no wonder months-long convalescences left some patients too weak to ever arise again.

One would like to think that this Victorian folly has faded into the oblivion it deserves, but I don't think so. Often the "decline" of the declining years — or even that more subtle crossing over from middle age to elderly — is hastened by an injury or illness that prompts both the sufferer and his sympathizers to advise "Oh, my dear, you must rest."

Many still believe that weakness after being bedridden for some time is a temporary disability from which the patient, *given sufficient rest*, will naturally recover. But recovery requires work, and exercise should be part of convalescence lest too much rest over too long a time permanently crank a person's level of activity down a notch or two.

Prescribing exercise has become routine when a person has had a heart attack or stroke, but what about the person who has had a gall bladder operation? A hysterectomy? A hernia repair? Or broken a rib, or been bruised in a traffic accident, or simply had a nasty bout of flu? If your doctor doesn't tell you to walk and work out as you recover, for your body's sake, ask.

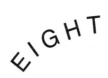

Posture with a Pillow on Your Head

When I was a kid, schools gave lessons in posture. They were formally part of gym class, along with calisthenics, but less formally they pervaded every class. "Get your elbows off the desk, Carol." "Hold in that tummy, George." "You're slumping, Mabel. Stand straight."

These admonitions were as frequent (and as ho-hum to us) as the reminder never to leave home without a handkerchief. We were told to pretend we were hanging by a string attached to the top of our skull, and we practiced walking with a dictionary on our head. Our teachers were exemplars: backs straight, heads high, shoulders back, bellies in. My school even gave an annual posture award. It usually went to a particular girl who looked like a ramrod and walked like a robot.

In retrospect, and with the conviction that I now know more about this subject than my teachers did, she should have gotten the award for Statue of the Year. By now, that stiff girl is probably frozen from the neck down. Posture isn't just the way you hold yourself when still, it's the way you move when you walk, bend, lean, and lift. It has to do with fluidity and balance. I imagine we were taught good posture with the aim of our becoming proper young ladies and gentlemen, but my goal is to spare your joints the crush of slumped positions and your muscles the rude shock of awkward movements.

Besides, you'll look younger.

Posture instructions always begin with the curve of the spine that proper posture is intended to promote. My posture and my spinal curve are exemplary. From the side, the spine curves forward just below the base of the skull, then gently back toward the shoulder blades, then an equal curve toward the belly, then a little flip back and down at the tail. The string of a plumb bob hung from the back of my skull touches the curve at my shoulder blades and the curve at the base of my spine. My ears are in line with my shoulders, my arms hang straight along my sides, and — the important mechanical principle here — the weight of a burden carried on my head would be distributed equally all along my backbone.

True, we don't carry water jugs, but the column of air above us weighs about 14 pounds per square inch of skull surface (over 1,100 pounds for the average pate), and the head itself weighs at least another 10 pounds. We carry that burden during all our waking hours even if we carry nothing else.

Each step we take knocks the spine from below as the foot hits the ground; the shock is the greater the heavier the walker and the faster the pace (and, of course, the less resilient the walking surface — hence we "pound the pavement"). Running smacks the foot with an impact two to three times the runner's weight at every step. This crunch is partly cushioned by the jelly-filled disks between the vertebrae, by the foot's arch, and by whatever elasticity there is in the knee and hip. But the spine's sinuous curve also gives the back just enough spring to help it absorb the shock of a jump or jog without squashing the disks too much.

While you're picturing this pleasant curve, you're probably holding your spine as true to the picture as you can, but stand up now and let yourself slump. There could be one of two things wrong with your standing posture. The more usual one is the gorilla stance. The head is forward, the upper back is humped, the curve at the small of the back is straightened, the arms hang in front of the thighs, and the

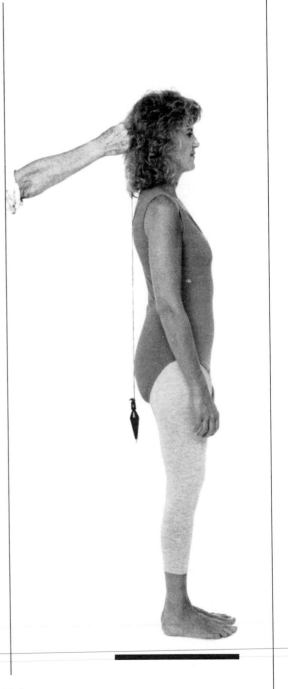

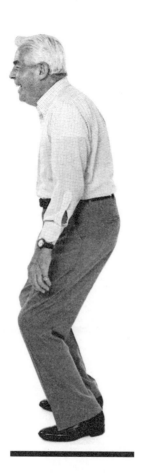

The gorilla stance

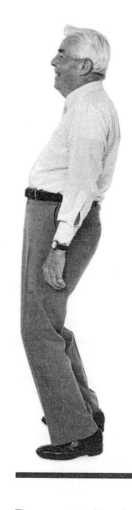

The pregnant-with-twins stance

knees are bent. Imagine a weight placed on the head now: The hump at the shoulders takes too much weight and bows beneath it, and the straight portion of the spine is scrunched.

The other possibility is that you're standing as though you were nine months pregnant with twins. Your belly's way out there; your chin juts forward; your hands hang too far to the rear. Your back's swayed in above the hips and out at the shoulders in an exaggerated curve. A load on your head would bend your back into an even deeper S-curve, pull your muscles, and squish your disks unevenly.

Don't run for the nearest bag of groceries to see what a load on your head might do to your back; that much weight could really hurt it. But walking around the house with a small floppy couch pillow, about fourteen inches square, on your head will show you what's wrong and help you get it right. A pillow isn't as heavy or as likely to fall as *Webster's New Collegiate*, but you'll feel the strain if your back is swayed in the middle or humped at the top. To balance the pillow, you'll naturally hold your abdomen in, your shoulders back, your chin tucked, and your head straight. Your spine will have no choice but to curve the way it ought to.

The pillow has to be a floppy one to stay on at all, and it shouldn't be slippery. If nothing handy fits the bill, use a folded blanket instead.

Try doing a few ordinary things with the pillow or blanket on your head. Answer the telephone. Sit down in an armchair. Get up. Set the table. Eat.

You'll find that all your movements are affected. You walk with a gliding motion, taking up the shift from leg to leg by bending a little at the hip lest the pillow slip sideways. To keep the pillow from falling forward when you place an object on the table, you bend a bit at the knee. You have to support your weight on the arms or seat of the chair to sit down as well as to stand up. You don't hunch a shoulder up to answer the telephone or to eat; you keep both shoulders down and level. All your movements are slower and smoother; less work is done by your back alone.

You'll also notice that walking with a pillow on your head is a stretching and toning exercise that you'll feel in whatever joints have been restricted or whatever muscles have been weakened by your slumped posture in the past. A few minutes each evening spent wearing a pillow like a crown will straighten you out considerably in time and make it easier to maintain better posture even under the light-headed conditions of everyday life.

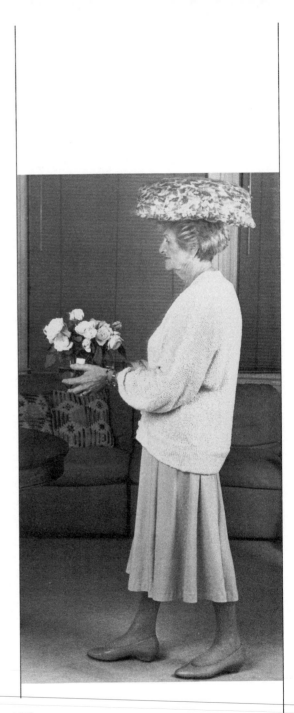

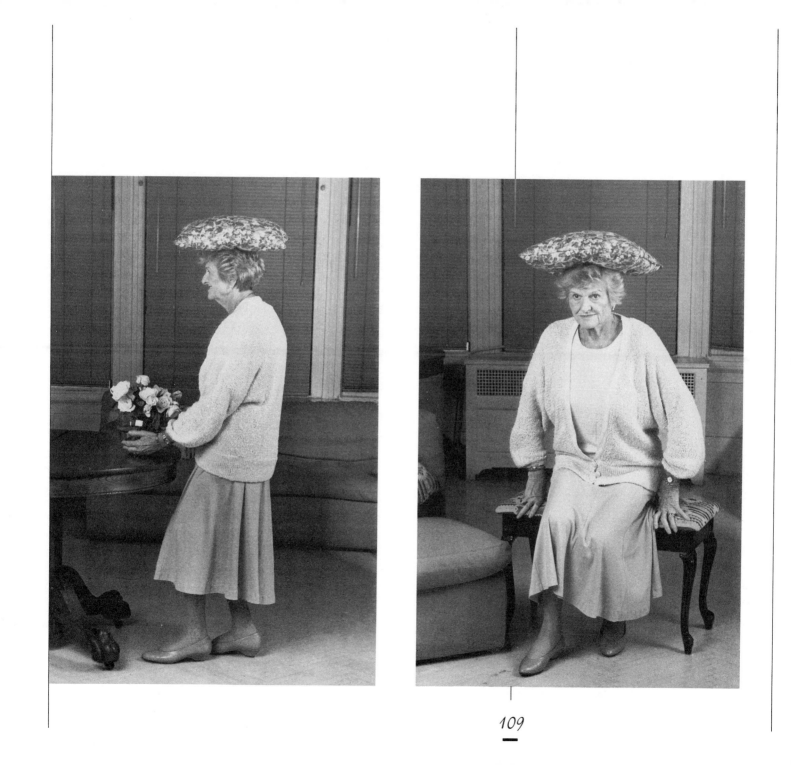

Everyday life is the issue here. Let's say you're building a barbecue in the backyard and you've bent to pick up bricks. What's bent? If the answer is your back alone, your back's not going to like it. If you think of the size of the thigh muscles in a leg of lamb compared to the puny tidbit of back muscle in a lamb chop, you'll realize that your legs can take a good deal more lifting than your back. So make them. Squat a little when you lift. That way your thigh muscles will share the work with your back muscles, and both will be the better for it.

A lift from a squat doesn't work if you're too far from what you're lifting — if you try, you'll fall on your nose. You have to get right above the load. That's a problem if the load is bags of groceries on the far side of the shopping cart or the bags that always seem to slide to the rear of the trunk. Pull the bags or cartons toward you before you lift them. Don't load heavy packages onto car seats or on the floor behind. There's no way you're going to get them out again with grace or safety. Here's a trick for bags that slip back in the car: Ask that groceries be put into plastic bags with handles. (Environmentalists prefer plastic grocery bags to paper ones because paper bags don't decay in landfills and are more bulky than plastic.) Hang the handles outside the car trunk and slam the lid on them. Your car will look a little frilly in the rear, but the bags will be at hand when you get home.

Wiping up spilt milk or picking up a golf ball from the green doesn't seem like much of a load on the back, but there are worse and better ways to reach down and straighten up again. The worst way is the way you're probably too stiff for, anyway: leaning without bending your knees. Even if you can do it, don't. The movement stretches the lower back muscles to their max, then asks them immediately to contract to pull the weight of your trunk to an upright position again. Again, flex the knees a bit. That keeps your center of gravity beneath your spine rather than in front of it, and the lift back up is shared by the thighs.

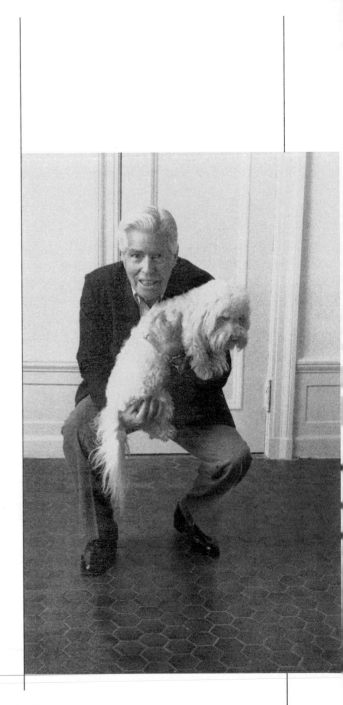

Another way to descend is to put one foot behind you as you bend your knees; you end up crouched somewhat like a runner readied for the gun. Your arms assist in getting up again: One hand pushes against the floor, the other against the bent knee.

Practice these bends whenever you can, such as when guests are coming and the Sunday paper is all over the floor, or after a child has littered the living room with toys, or the lamp's unplugged, or the corner of the rug is flipped up, or you've dropped a pocketful of change.

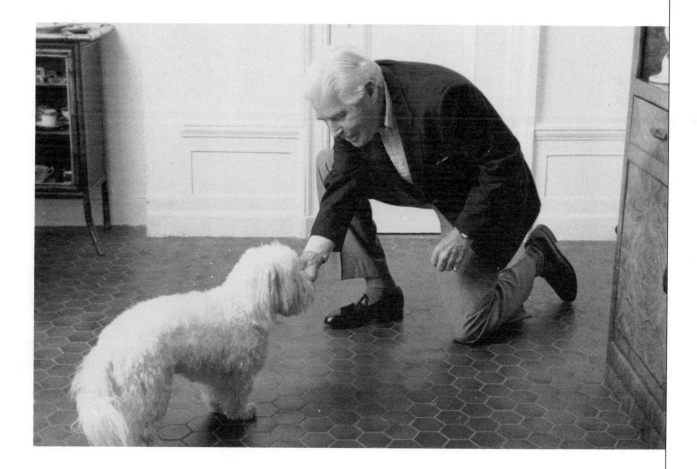

Everyone who gardens is down on their hands and knees often and, unless they like to crawl from weed to weed, must often get up as well. If they can. If their back doesn't clutch and their knees don't crack. My co-author, who positively enjoys grubbing in the dirt, is old enough to know exactly what I mean, so I've shown her how to avoid getting stuck on all fours in the soil. With your arms, you "walk" yourself back into a squat, then straighten your back slowly. That uncricks that part of the aging anatomy. Then you put one knee on the ground and, leaning forward, push with one hand on the ground and the other on your knee to slowly lift yourself upright. The knee may still make a popping noise, but you will get up. The longer you stay down on all fours, the harder it is to get back on two feet.

That's true of any posture: Hold it too long, and you'll look as if you're playing the child's game called Statue. I locked my own neck the other night by spending an hour and a half immobile, gripped by a television drama. My advice to myself, and to you too, is to change position every few minutes.

Sometimes circumstances trap you in one posture for hours, such as when you're belted into the driver's seat on a long trip. A country doctor in Maine has come up with a swell solution for keeping the neck and shoulders on the move while driving. He turns on the radio to a symphony and conducts the orchestra with his nose. I find a car with cruise control very helpful; it frees your feet from the pedals. Certainly you should stop the car more often than you used to. Move (stretch!) and change the position of the seat to a little higher or lower and tilt it at a slightly different angle. Headrests are handy for pressing your head against to stretch the back of your neck — an exercise you don't even have to wait for a red light to do.

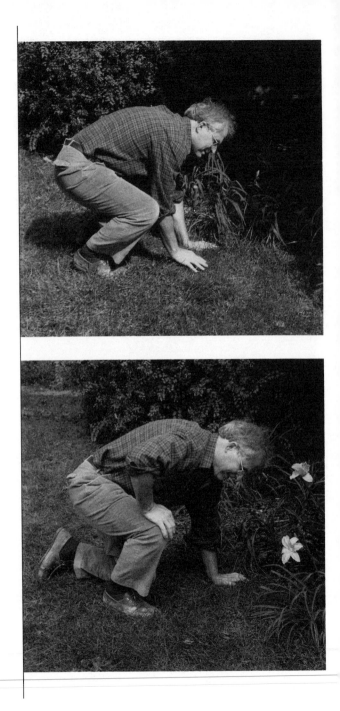

Glasses can be an insidious body cramper, especially bifocals and trifocals and the continuous curve lenses that are an alternative. A friend of mine who uses her computer a lot discovered that she was tilting her head back to see the screen because the middle portion of her trifocals was too low, and her neck was really hurting. However, when she had a new pair of glasses made to correct the problem, she found that seeing the road when driving was a problem. Neither pair was right for golf because she saw the ball at the end of her club through lenses designed for a book held close or a screen at arm's length. To see through the top portion, designed for greater distance, she had to putt with her chin on her chest.

All such glasses blur steps, curbs, broken sidewalks, and the rutted path beneath the wearer's feet, and they lead, I'm sure, to tense posture, hesitant steps, and accidents. I can't think of a solution other than several pairs of glasses. It's something to talk about with your eye doctor.

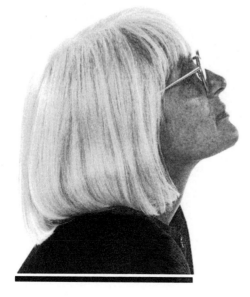

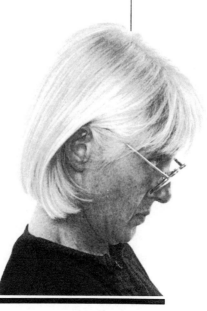

I'm convinced that handedness causes crooked postures that often lead to trouble. Jobs such as hauling in a fishing net or pushing a wheelbarrow work both sides of the body evenly, but people write and draw with their right or left hand, and that may throw off their whole body symmetry. Some architects and engineers stand at their drafting table for hours with one hip cocked and the opposite leg bent, thus placing all their weight on the cocked hip and the straight leg below it and all the pressure on that side of the back. You can imagine that standing with the spine curved sideways all day is not good, but they can't switch hips because the choice of which hip sticks out has to do with which hand they draw with. They're leaning on the other hand,

Electric Wrist

The tendons that flex fingers run through a structure called the carpal tunnel, a small space between the eight bones of the wrist and the bracelet of ligament that encircles them. The sensory nerves of the fingers also run through the carpal tunnel. As you move your fingers, the tendons slide back and forth beneath the ligament bracelet. Continual sliding abrades both tendons and ligament, inflaming them until they press against the nerves that share the tunnel. The symptoms from pressed nerves are numbness in the fingers and stabs of pain in the wrist that feel like electric shocks.

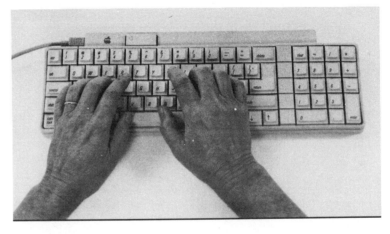

This syndrome is caused by repetitive motions such as typing. In the old days of manual machines, the typist had to pull the carriage return at the end of every line, insert a piece of paper at the end of every page, and stop periodically to correct an error. These frequent changes of motion gave the wrists a break. Computers have made it possible to type for long hours without respite. To the typist, keyboarding feels effortless compared to banging out the pages on an ancient Remington, but the tendons and ligaments need frequent rests to repair themselves, and computers have not been easy on them.

which is no good for that shoulder. Obviously, the neck is out of kilter too. So should they sit on a stool?

One of my patients, an architect, had a chronically inflamed elbow from leaning it on the table while he drew, and he sat on a stool. An editor I treated had pinched a nerve in her neck by leaning her head on one hand while marking manuscripts with the other. Even idle games may involve occupational hazards. I heard on television about a thirty-five-year-old woman who developed painful tendonitis in the wrist she used to play Nintendo for five hours nonstop.

Use stretches as a diagnostic tool. If one side of your neck or hip or back feels stiffer than the other when you stretch it, or if one portion of your body seems harder to move than others, suspect that a posture you assume for hours during the day is to blame. Think it out. From top to bottom. Where's your head? It shouldn't be tilted to one side or hanging over the desk. Where are your shoulders? If you're writing memos, one is likely to be higher than the other. Holding the telephone to your ear with a shoulder is a common sin. Get a speakerphone. If you always sit in the same corner of the couch, the same elbow is always propped on the arm. Try the other side for a change. One writer I know not only crosses one leg over the other while she types but also wraps her ankles so her legs are twisted like a licorice stick. Imagine!

Only the closest questioning revealed that the photographer who came to me for her aching back had for thirty years carried her heavy gear slung on her right shoulder, never on her left. People dig right-footed, or hoe right-handed, and never think to shift for a few minutes now and then. In which hand do you carry a suitcase, on which hip a child? Which foot, which hand, is forward as you vacuum? Shift! Such shifts feel awkward at first, but even lifelong habits can be altered, and a straighter posture, a more balanced bend, and a more equitable distribution of load can become habitual in time.

That writer who twists her legs also hunches her shoulders as though she were a vulture grappling with the carcass of her keyboard. Naturally, she hurts.

I tell her, get a new chair.

The same applies to you if you sit down while you work and it hurts, and if your boss can be made to see the wisdom of spending money for a new chair now instead of for your disability in the future. You're supposed to sit with your back just slightly curved; your head should be in line with your hips and shoulders, not the keyboard. Your shoulders should hang limp as you work; your hands should be level with your elbows. All this is impossible for the writer in her present torture chamber. Her chair is too low, so she has to lift her shoulders to type. The seat is so deep, its edge hits her at the knee; she twists her legs to prop them higher. The chair might as well be backless, for what back there is stands a good 6 inches from her own. Chairs ought to be more like car seats, curved to fit the human shape from knee to butt, from butt to shoulder blade.

I wonder if all furniture designers are over 6 feet tall. Why else would chairs and couches have such deep seats? From my tailbone to the back of my knee is about 17 inches. The seat of an average easy chair is 22 inches. The only way to sit in such a chair is to slump. The blithe suggestion to place a pillow at the small of the back is no help if there are still inches of air behind the shoulders. And chair and sofa arms are often too high: They push the shoulder up, pressing the ball to the socket.

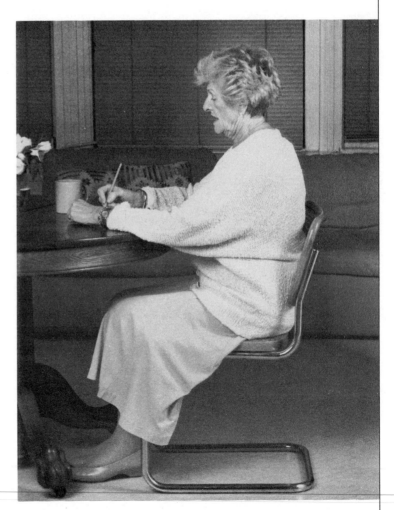

Six-footers must design desks and tables, too. An ordinary wooden chair seat is 18 inches off the floor; desks and table surfaces are 29 inches high. That puts my elbow 3 inches lower than my hand; to write, I have to prop my right elbow up, which pushes my body to the left, which forces me to lean on the other elbow to support my tilted head. That's how that editor hurt her neck. Such a lean could just as easily injure the elbow, too.

In a perfect world, furniture would come in sizes, small, medium, and large. Chairs and couches would be contoured snugly to the human form. In this imperfect world, one has to shop around a lot to find anything designed for proper posture in a size that fits. But I do suggest — modestly, because I'm talking money here — that at least your work area and your favorite relaxing chair be furniture that fits.

No matter how comfortably seated, you shouldn't sit for more than thirty minutes at a time. Get up, walk around, stretch. Muscles tensed in the same position for a long time constrict their own blood supply and may cramp. That's what causes stiff necks and writer's cramp. The same thing happens to backs, just from sitting still. The leg-twisting writer found herself bound to her chair by a knot in her lower back one afternoon. The old chair. The one I warned her about.

Sleep Without Slump

Well, you may be thinking, time for a nap. Watch out. There are better and worse ways to sleep, too. Lying down is a posture.

Reclining on a couch or sleeping in a bed doesn't necessarily put the body in a relaxed position. A snooze on a sofa snuggled in a pile of pillows slumps the neck, humps the shoulders, and pulls the sway right out of the lower back. A night's sleep on a mushy mattress with a tough pillow underneath the head does the same. Both are bad. Sleeping on the stomach is even worse. The neck is twisted too far; the back is arched too much.

Dream Paralysis

A common dream that almost everyone has had involves an inability to move. You must answer the telephone but can't reach for it; you have to catch a train but can't run to it. A similar experience is that of trying to awaken from a bad dream but finding yourself unable to move a muscle.

These experiences are real. During dreaming, the skeletal muscles are paralyzed. Although they may twitch occasionally, like those of a dreaming dog, the coordinated movement required for reaching or walking isn't possible. This is a necessary precaution. The cortex of the brain, the seat of consciousness, intellect, and sensory awareness, is as fully active during dreaming as during our waking hours. Were we able to move, we might enact our dreams, and that would certainly be dangerous.

During ordinary sleep, the cortex is shut down, but our muscles are quite capable of tossing and turning us, slapping at mosquitoes, or scratching where they bite.

When you lie down, your spine should be curved in just the same way it is when you stand up. That's not possible in the reclined position people take to doze on the couch after dinner or read mysteries in bed. To keep the curve when lying on your back, use one pillow under your head and another under your knees. A hard pillow can raise the head too high; use a soft one. You can also keep a good sleeping posture by lying on your side with one knee drawn up and a pillow under your head; some people are more comfortable with both knees bent, with a small pillow between them.

If, when you sit on the bed amid magazines and snacks, everything falls into the well your weight creates, the surface is too springy and too soft. Firm it up with three-quarter-inch interior plywood, cut to fit by the lumberyard, slipped between the mattress and the spring. You don't really need springs at all. An excellent combination of "mattress" and "spring" is a thick futon over plywood. Futons are stuffed with cotton and have no springs. When you lie on a futon, it conforms to your body's curves, hollowing at the hips and shoulders, humping in between. Over time, a futon develops a kind of custom fit that's remarkably comfortable and gives excellent support.

In fact, if you opt for this radical departure from Beauty Rest, I can offer you a reward beyond your wildest dreams: I'll let you do your floor exercises in bed.

The All-over Ache

That ache-all-over feeling some people have when they awaken is a sign of a sedentary life. The fancy medical term for this aching is hypokinesis syndrome. Hypokinesis means lack of motion. Syndrome means that many things are awry, such as scant circulation to muscles, meager food storage in the muscles, shortened muscles, weak muscles, poorly lubricated joints, and fibers in the tendons and ligaments that are adhering to the joints and to each other.

Some people ache only in the winter and blame it on the cold. Some ache after they've been bedridden with an illness and blame it on the flu. Sooner or later, most everybody blames it on their age. But immobility — seasonal, medical, or otherwise — is always the cause, and movement is always the cure.

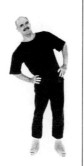

NINE

Work: A Vacation from Exercise

Exercise is work, but it's not like real work. Real work rewards you with real things: tomatoes you've grown, shelves you've built, rooms you've painted. More strength per muscle and more motion per joint are real in their way, but they don't taste like a fresh tomato.

Exercise is intellectually dull; work is not. You don't think about exercise when you're planting the corn. You concentrate on hoeing a straight row, you calculate the probable date of harvest, you imagine butter melting over the crop's sweet fat ears sometime in August. That imagery has got to be more gripping than thoughts of firming up your tummy. A person unloading boards from the station wagon is aiming to get them into the garage, not to strengthen his back and biceps. A person hanging wallpaper is making the guest room gorgeous. Sure, he's making muscles too, but how can that bore him if he's not even thinking about it?

When you're lying on the floor doing stretches, there's nothing to look at but the ceiling, nothing to smell but carpet dust, nothing to listen to but your own breathing or maybe the morning news. So you want a vacation from exercise? Work!

Gardening probably offers the best overall workout a body can get. It involves plenty of walking, not just behind a mower but to get the rake you forgot to load into the wheelbarrow and the bag of peat moss that wouldn't fit in on the first trip. Then you have to make another trip to carry the flats from the porch, then to drag the hose, then to haul the weeds to the compost heap, and then to put everything away at the end of the afternoon. That's natural aerobics, and think of the air! It beats sucking up exhaust fumes on a city sidewalk.

Gardening is what physical therapists call low-impact exercise. It doesn't bang the knees or wrench the shoulders or slam an elbow out of joint. Each task uses a large set of muscles. Pushing a wheelbarrow or a mower uses the muscles of chest and arms, legs and hips, and the whole back. Pruning with loppers uses the upper body — hands to shoulders, chest to back. Grunt work like digging is great for the belly as well as the back. Raking and hoeing work out the arms. When you garden, you lift, drag, push, pull. You stretch to lop a high branch from the apple tree, stoop to cut a sucker from the pear, crouch to sow the carrot seeds, twist the hips to reach for a bulb in the sack beside you, swivel a shoulder to retrieve the pruners from your back pocket, arch the back to firm the soil around a rose.

A special advantage of gardening is that it involves continual switching from one task to another. Frequent changes of position, and shifting the work from one set of muscles to another, let some joints and muscles relax and recover while others get a workout. There's less fatigue, and less chance of an injury or later soreness, than if you worked for the same amount of time on just one type of task. In fact, the recuperation advantage in switching among tasks lets you work for more hours and so get more exercise and lose more calories. A person weighing 150 pounds expends about 400 calories by spending twenty minutes each at mowing, weeding, pruning, and raking. Not to mention the work accomplished and the rewards thereof!

The Cunning of the Craft

Many people take up gardening for the first time in their retirement and find it harder than they had anticipated. Here is some advice for older gardeners who have not yet learned the cunning of the craft.

Sharpen your shovels. They're supposed to *cut* through soil. Don't ask a shovel, or the knees that push it, to jam through roots. Use loppers for that. Hone your loppers frequently. Dull loppers wrench shoulders. Hoes should be sharp too, unless you want your arms to drop with exhaustion in ten minutes and your back to bring you to the ground. Don't grapple with stones. That's what a crowbar is for. Bend your knees when lifting potted plants. And don't wrestle heavy bags of fertilizer, bales of peat moss, or balled and burlapped plants into the wheelbarrow. Turn the barrow on its side, roll or drag the burden into it, then right it by pulling and leaning on the wheelbarrow's opposite edge. Work at an unhurried and deliberate pace. If you find yourself working too fast, and so tiring too quickly, hum a slow tune to slow yourself down.

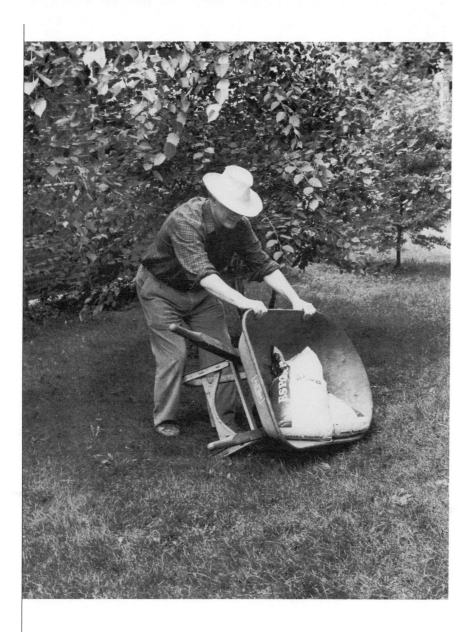

Certainly fitness and fatness are incompatible, and often a person determined to become fit decides to combine an exercise regime with a crash diet.

Crash diets, however, are most unwise. Exercise makes muscle fibers more efficient, and that's what you want them to be; dieting does the same for fat cells, but that's not what you want at all. When the body is suddenly deprived of food, it assumes there is a famine and permanently adjusts its metabolism to prepare for periods of starvation that may recur. Food is metabolized more completely, and fat cells educated by starvation store up more fat as insurance against lean times to come. After the crash diet is over, these efficiencies result in more fat from less food, and so you gain weight more easily than you did before.

The only way to trick this system is to avoid sounding the famine alarm. Eat smaller portions and leaner foods (fats and oils have by far the most calories per gram), but don't panic your fat by losing more than half a pound of it per week.

Much as gardening is an exercise expert's ideal of the perfect workout, it does have one major disadvantage: Unless you live in the most favorable climate, gardening is seasonal. Bounding up one fine March morning to plant potatoes after six months of being a couch potato yourself isn't smart. So — back to exercise. Yes, you should keep up those stretches and strengtheners during the long, dull months of winter, and yes, you weekend gardeners, you should do your trunk stretches before setting forth to turn the soil.

An even more severe drawback to gardening is that we city slickers have no place to do it. House plants don't require sweating; a patio planting is too small for physical challenge; even a backyard may demand too little work to call a workout. And what if you hate dirt beneath your fingernails?

Make a list of all the things you do in your life that could fall into the category of physical labor. The list may include shopping, cleaning, home repairs and maintenance, and a hobby such as carpentry. Now make a second list of all the things you have others do for you. That list, too, might include cleaning, shopping (if you have many things delivered), and home repair and maintenance. Now make a third list of the labor-saving devices you use, such as a vacuum cleaner, ride 'em mower, dishwasher, electric can opener, circular saw — even cars and elevators. Could you amend these lists to squeeze more work into your life?

To most people these days, the idea of squeezing work into, rather than out of, their lives is unnatural, if not downright subversive. We live in the age of convenience, when labor saved is leisure earned. But think about it. Opening a can with an electric can opener does not save time and does cost money. Opening a can with a manual opener is free and, depending on whether you have a twist-type hand opener or a wall-mounted one, exercises either your wrist or your shoulder. Vacuums are indeed better than brooms for thorough cleaning, but think of the small jobs — the cracker crumbs and doorway dirt. Sweep-

Warm Up or Cramp Up

The "warm" in warm-up is to be taken literally. Stretches and other exercises warm muscles and tendons by the friction of their own motion and by the increased blood flow that motion demands. As you may remember from science classes, heat speeds up chemical reactions. Chemical reactions within a warmed muscle fiber are also speeded up. The muscle takes in more food, extracts more energy from it, and responds more readily and smoothly to signals to contract. A cool muscle, by comparison, is not prepared to work. When suddenly put upon, it may cramp or tear. Tendons require warmth and gentle stretching for maximum flexibility. Warming up protects them, too, from tearing.

ing is a great movement for your hips and back and shoulders. How about the stretches involved in washing windows? Why give someone else the precious exercise you could have yourself?

A recent article in the *New York Times* bid an official farewell to spring cleaning. No one does it anymore, the article claimed; people have no time for unpacking stuffed closets, taking down dusty drapes, and doing all the shaking, scouring, scrubbing, and polishing that used to be a rite of spring. But look at it this way: If you're spending a couple of hours a week exercising (and especially if you've been spending money for the privilege), you could trade a month of boring routines for four weeks of spring cleaning and earn, in addition to body mainte-nance, a sparkling home and the clean conscience of having contrib-uted — through Goodwill Industries, for example — things you don't need that someone else can use. How's that for exercising both body and soul!

No fooling, if you're under eighty and not ill, you probably can paint your bathroom. You've never done it before? Neither have all those other people for whom how-to books are published. Jobs like painting are similar to gardening in that they involve the whole body in a full range of movements and postures. I do draw the line at house painting. I've had too many patients who have fallen off ladders.

Lots of city folks would like to have a dog but think it would be too much work to walk Rover three times a day. Consider this: a dog out merely to relieve himself needs five minutes only (less for a female). That's two walks, but hardly work. A dog out for exercise as well as toileting needs a good half hour's walk, the same as you do.

That's it, city folks: your daily dose of aerobics, and you get a dog to boot.

Every little dividend of effort you can add to the everyday chores of life adds to the total fitness profit you can reap and subtracts from the time you have to spend on exercise routines. Don't look for the nearest parking space. Park in the rear of the lot. You'll walk farther, and haul farther, to your body's general benefit. People who have to go from floor to floor where they work can use stairs instead of elevators.

The Company Dogs Keep

Strangers don't simply go up to one another on the street and say hello. But strangers greet dogs they've never met before with amazing outpourings of camaraderie: "My, look what we have here, such a beautiful fellow you are! I bet you'd love to chase those pigeons. What's your name, you gorgeous thing?" This lack of embarrassment when addressing a dog — this assumption of intimacy, this full-blown friendliness — leads naturally to conversation between stranger and dog owner that otherwise would be unthinkable. A number of serious studies have recorded the results: People who walk dogs meet more people, spend more time chatting, and make more friends around the neighborhood than those who walk alone.

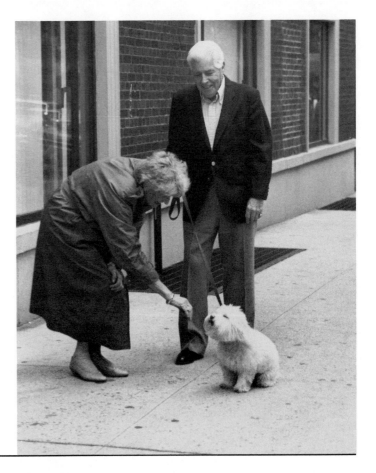

If your lawn is small, it's no big deal to push a reel mower through it, and you'll be sparing the world an unnecessary whiff of pollution too.

There's irony in the exercise business. Rowing machines mimic the action of rowing a rowboat, cycling machines mimic the action of pedaling a bike. People pay to own or use these stationary machines while actually getting to where they're going by gas-powered vehicles — and on top of that they worry about polluted air and their capacity to breathe, and so throw in an aerobics class as well. Get a boat, get a bike. Walk.

But what if you're eighty? It would be flippant and cruel to suggest to the truly venerable that spryness can be regained and strength rejuvenated by scrubbing the oven, hopping on a bike, or lugging bags of bone meal to the yard. At any level of activity, however, a person can put forth just a little more effort than is comfortable. As people stiffen with age, as their joints become arthritic and their muscles thin, they tend to spare themselves the discomfort of reaching to a shelf, stooping to the floor, carrying the groceries. They shop once a week instead of twice.

Each of these labor-saving decisions seems insignificant in itself, yet they add up. Elderly people often end up making life too convenient for their own good. They keep the few dishes they use daily out on the counter, where they needn't stretch to reach them; place next to a favorite chair all the things they could possibly want once they sit down, including a telephone and the remote control for the TV; place all their house plants on one stand so that they needn't walk to water them. The easier they make things for themselves, the weaker and stiffer they become, until the convenience that was originally an option becomes a necessity and life is spent sitting in a chair.

At any age, the principle is the same: Keep moving, keep working. If you can walk to the TV, get rid of that remote. Don't put that telephone extension on the table at your elbow. Don't group the plants. Feed the cat on the floor, not the counter; you need those several extra stoops a day. Reach the dishes up to the shelves where they belong, and put some of the things you need most often as high as you can stretch. Don't accept the neighbors' offers to take out your trash. Do accept their offers to take you shopping, and carry what you can.

Helplessness Is Hazardous to Your Health

It's well known that women tend to live longer than men. What's less well known is that men's mortality rate climbs steeply during the first year of retirement. That's a fact. How this special vulnerability of men is to be interpreted is more problematical, but researchers' best judgment so far is that men aren't prepared to keep themselves employed around the house. They feel useless, helpless, overwhelmed, and depressed. People under such stress produce an excess of stress hormones: adrenaline and cortisone. Adrenaline taxes the heart and raises blood pressure. Heart attacks and strokes become more likely. Cortisone depresses the immune system, so infections can take hold; so can cancer.

You men who are reading this, I'm not saying it to scare you; I think that fitness in your case includes something more Darwinian than is the case with women: fitness in the sense of adaptation to the particular environment of home. I think a better adaptation is possible. I think you can become more fit for what may face you in the future, and that if you do, you will be less at risk.

Men of our generation weren't taught as boys to cook, clean, launder, sew, or shop. They are seldom aware that a home must be run — scheduled, organized, managed, maintained, and continually inventoried. They know a lot about interpersonal relations at their workplace, but not necessarily about interpersonal relations with plumbers, fuel companies, shopkeepers, neighbors, and community organizations. They think there's nothing to do at home; if they do realize that there's work to be done, they don't know how to do it.

This year one man I know retired from his job at the age of sixty-five. His wife is the world's worst cook, and knows it. He hates her cooking. He hates the kitchen wallpaper. So does his wife. She complains about the yard, the straggly shrubs, the lilacs choked with suckers. He agrees. But his biggest complaint, and the one that's really getting him down, is that he has nothing to do.

You get the point.

For both sexes, keeping busy, feeling able, doing work, participating in the community, are positive protections against illness and enfeeblement. Maybe endorphins, the pleasure-giving chemicals that reward activity and effort, are responsible for the generally greater vigor and enthusiasm of those who, despite aches and creaks and the approach of their ninth decade, plant pansies and prepare picnics for their annual Fourth of July family reunion. The wonderful old lady whose pansies and picnics I'm thinking of was named Citizen of the Year by the civic organization of her hometown when she was ninety-one. Now, at ninety-four, she still works for the organization. Her job is to lick stamps. "Well," she says, with her usual flair for exaggeration, "I can't see, I can't hear, I can't walk, but there's nothing wrong with my tongue!" Or, by the way, with her blood pressure, cholesterol level, mind, or heart.

Not to mention her spirit.

Relax!

I'll never forget the day I walked into the office to find my eight-o'clock patient tensely pacing the floor. "I make a point of being early for my appointments," he barked, "and I expect those I deal with to do the same." Then he asked for my qualifications.

I didn't have to ask what ailed him. This man was a battering ram. He led with his head through doors, into people, as though to bulldoze his way in the world. He was a lawyer, his specialty was corporate takeovers, and he had squashed his own disks by the force of his own tensed neck muscles.

People carry more than the weight of gravity on their shoulders. They carry heavy ambitions, pressing obligations, and a heap of worry. The posture of this man — his jaw thrust, shoulders hunched, and head jutting — was the same as that a Neanderthal might have taken when threatened by a Cro-Magnon: It's a defensive posture, a protective duck from danger that also readies the fists to punch. An irritated boss or an overdue assignment isn't like the danger cave men faced, but the primitive part of the brain that runs the shoulder hunch isn't clever at distinguishing shades of meaning. But what was I to say to him? Relax?

I can't stand it when people tell me to relax. If they were paying my rent, I could relax. If they were both paying my bills and taking care of my patients, I could goof off, have a beer, go to the zoo, or read

Muscles Need Vacations

A tired muscle is one that has accumulated waste products and needs time off to get rid of them. Sleep isn't necessary for that. The brain needs sleep, but muscles recuperate through rest alone and get no special benefit from your night's dreamings. They take their rest — and shuck their wastes — quickly when you shift from one motion or position to another for a while or when you relax for half an hour or so. Your body will feel much less tired by the evening if you give your muscles a variety of short vacations all through the day.

128

the comics. Relaxing isn't a command performance; tensions aren't shucked as easily as a camper slips off a backpack. You have to find ways to wriggle out from under. It may not be easy; learning to relax can take work. But if exercise is one side of the coin you pay to stay younger longer, relaxation is the other.

Hands On for Relaxation

I was interested to read that babies won't grow unless they're stroked. Stroking the naked skin directly affects both the efficiency of metabolism and the rate at which the baby's own growth hormone is doled out. A baby who isn't fondled can't use the food he or she eats, and remains puny in spite of the excellence of every other element of care. I haven't read of similar research on the physiological effects of stroking grown-ups, but massage therapists, who spend hours daily massaging knotted muscles, are convinced that their patients are eased more deeply

Sex with an Aching Back

Nothing — no massage, no stroke, no visit to a physical therapist — relaxes every muscle in the body as thoroughly as sex. But those with chronic backache often fear that sex will give them painful spasms, and such deprivation makes them all the more depressed and tense.

Sex doesn't have to be athletic; why should it even be copulation? Surely at our age we know sensualities that we had no idea of when our backs grappled more violently with adolescent urges and the need to reproduce.

A comfortable position is supine with a folded towel beneath the small of the back and a pillow below the knees. A comfortable approach is the slow, patient, generous, and sensuous sex that we've learned with intimacy and age and that doesn't necessarily extend to penetration. The point is orgasm, the quintessential stroke that leaves us limp as an infant, even to the knotted muscles of the back.

than their muscles go. Our own senses attest to the fact that massages, rubdowns, hugs — and yes, sex too — are emotionally soothing as well as muscularly relaxing.

Local benefit from massage is well understood. Pressured stroking mechanically eases tight muscles and keeps fibers from adhering in the joints. Blood flow increases as muscles ease their grip and as heat from friction expands capillary walls. Increased blood flow speeds healing. Massage also reduces pain, in two ways. More relaxed and better oxygenated muscles hurt less, and the sensation of rubbing along the surface of the skin blocks pain coming from deeper in the tissues.

Massage is a skill well worth learning. Sometimes you can practice it on yourself. More often you can use it to relax somebody else. There are basic mechanical principles involved: Your body must be in a position to exert considerable pressure without discomfort to yourself, and your partner's body must be supported so that he or she remains relaxed in spite of the pressure you're applying. For example, you can't lean your hands into a person's back muscles from the side; you haven't enough leverage from that position, you can't exert force evenly to both sides of the back, and your imbalanced posture will tire you quickly. You also can't give a back rub to someone who is sitting because he or she would have to tense up to resist the pressure of your hands. Massage therapists work standing with their patient lying down on a small, padded table, but you can make do with other positions suggested here. Although I'll give you pictures and descriptions to get you started, the experience of what works to relax a partner will teach you more. None of these examples is for medical therapy to injured joints and muscles. They're to be used for relaxation only.

Back rub: A back rub can be done with your partner lying face down on the floor and you kneeling or with your partner lying crosswise on a bed and you standing. Your hands should glide easily over the skin. Use a lubricant, such as baby oil, body lotion, or liniment.

Stand or kneel behind your partner's head. Use both hands, fingers together, and lean your weight into the heels of your hands. First place your hands on both sides of the spine at the neck and glide them downward along the large muscles of the back all the way to the base of the spine. Then move your hands apart and glide them back up again along the sides of the back, inward along the shoulder muscles, back to the neck where you began.

Repeat this circling glide rhythmically for several minutes without lifting your hands and pressing hard on the downward stroke, lightly on the return.

Neck and shoulder massage: For this one, your partner sits in a chair and you stand behind him. Because your hands won't be moving very far, you don't need to use a lubricant, although you may if you prefer.

Support your partner's head by placing one hand at his forehead. With the other hand, grasp the muscles at the base of the skull and, while pressing quite hard, knead them between thumb and fingers. Move down along the ridge of the muscles a little at a time until you've reached the shoulders.

No special support is needed to massage the shoulder muscles as long as your partner is comfortably seated. Standing directly behind him, grasp the muscles to both sides of the neck and squeeze them between your thumb and fingers. Press your thumbs into the flesh and move them in a circular, kneading motion. Gradually shift your hands outward until you've massaged the muscles all the way from the neck to the edge of the shoulders.

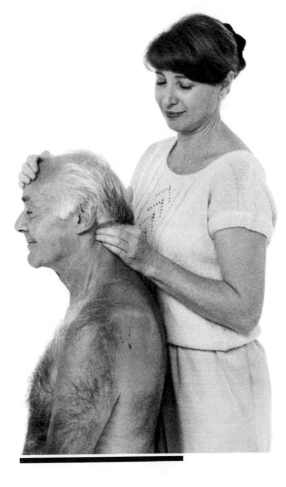

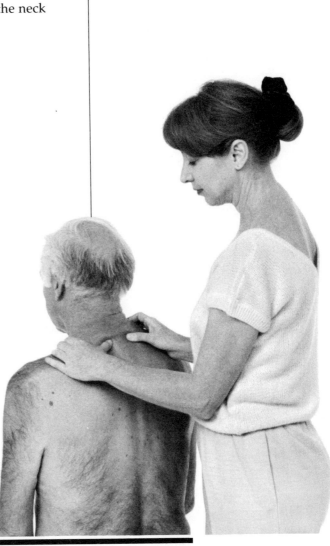

132

Head and face massage: This massage relaxes the facial muscles and improves circulation in the scalp. It is often used to relieve tension headaches.

Your partner lies down for this one, and you kneel behind his head. Start with the scalp, doing one side at a time. Support his head with one hand; with the other, press your fingertips to the scalp behind the ear and move them in a circular motion, as if you were giving a shampoo. Still pressing and circling, creep gradually up the skull to the hairline, out to the temple, and back down behind the ear to where you began, shifting the supporting hand as necessary so that your partner never has to resist the pressure with his own muscles. Then switch hands and massage the other side of the skull.

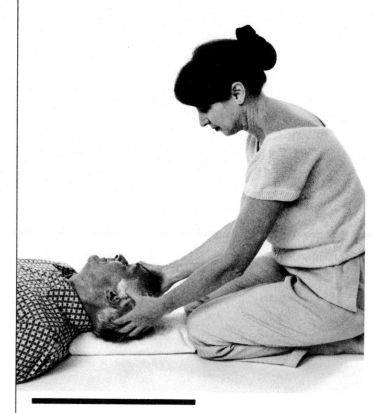 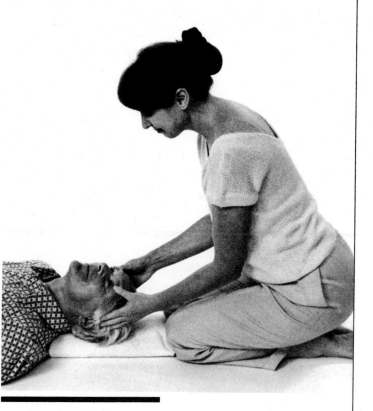

Use both hands to massage the brow and temples. Your spread fingers support your partner's head on both sides. Press your thumbs into his eyebrows to both sides of his nose and slowly stroke, still pressing, out toward the temples. Repeat for a minute or so. Then shift your hands down a bit so that your thumbs are at his temples. Press your thumbs in and massage the temples with a circular motion.

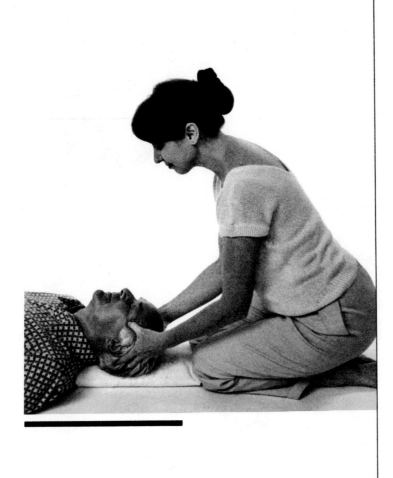

Hand and foot massage: A lubricant is really necessary for massaging the feet and hands.

Support your partner's hand with both your hands beneath it, and spread it open by holding his thumb down with your thumb. Use your other thumb to massage the palm in a circular, kneading motion. Then massage along the channels between the finger bones: Squeeze each channel in turn between your thumb and fingers, and walk your fingers along it from wrist to finger web. The wrist and finger lifts on pp. 100–101 may be included in a hand massage.

Finish the massage with a finger stretch: Support the hand at the wrist. Grasp the fingers one by one between your thumb and index finger and pull toward you gently, letting your grip slide all the way from the base of the finger

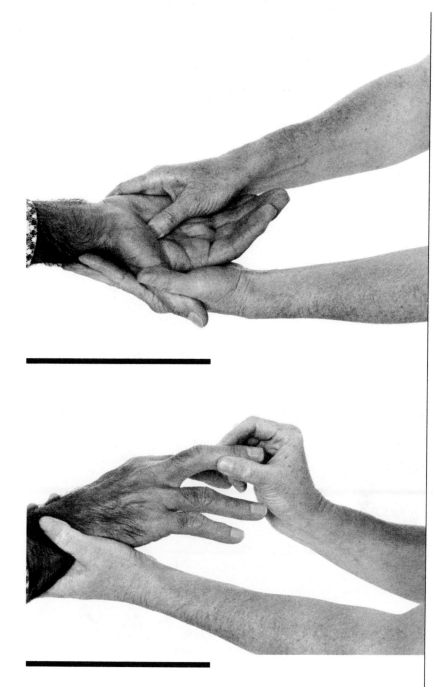

to the fingertip. Foot massage is similar. Hold your partner's foot in both hands and use your thumbs to knead along the arch and ball. Support the foot under the heel to gently spread and stretch each toe. Bending each toe upward feels good, too.

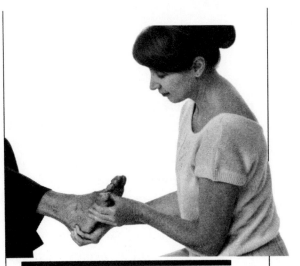

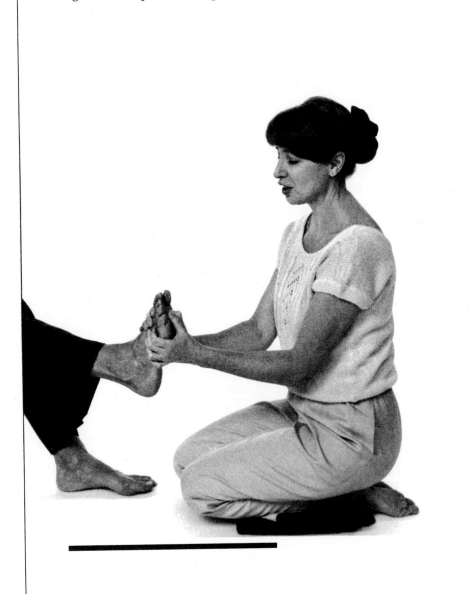

I know a family of Tibetan Buddhists who meditate for twenty minutes every morning, all three generations of them, down to the ten-year-old child. They find meditation indispensable for facing the day with equanimity. I had a tense patient in her sixties who sought, and found, tranquillity through yoga. Other patients have benefited from biofeedback relaxation therapy. A friend relaxes himself by stitching needlepoint. Walking relaxes me.

All these methods of relaxation work. Everything from knitting to chanting works. There must, therefore, be some common denominator among the techniques, religious and secular, by which the mind finds calmness and the body can relax.

All such relaxations take the mind off the self and let it sail. People who relax by stitching, meditating, walking, and praying all describe the same phenomenon: a sort of mental drifting as though one were outside oneself. That mental state, alert but not self-involved, is most usually achieved through some repetitive and rhythmic activity, whether the chanting of a mantra, the click of knitting needles, or a repeated footfall on the street.

If you've found your own technique for letting your mind run free, you ought to do it routinely, setting aside a special time each day as the Tibetan family does for meditation. Knowing a relaxation routine doesn't help if you don't practice it regularly, just like an exercise routine.

For those who haven't hit on a method of their own (as was certainly the case with the tense corporate lawyer), there are many courses available in stress control and relaxation. Some have an Eastern flavor; others, such as biofeedback, emanate from the Western discipline of behavioral psychology. Which you choose is a matter of personality. The corporate lawyer chose biofeedback for its more technological approach. You may also learn a craft.

No matter what you choose, the technique may not be relaxing

How Biofeedback Works

As skeletal muscles contract, they produce electrical signals like those the heart produces as it beats. Heartbeats are measured electrically with an electrocardiograph machine, which detects the varying strength and frequency of heart muscle signals and records them as a graph. A biofeedback machine is similar but less intimidating. It has only two electrodes — those suction cups that are stuck to the skin with jelly — and they are usually placed on the forearm, not all over the body. A biofeedback machine records the level of the muscles' electrical activity by a light or sound display rather than on a printed tape.

During relaxation therapy, you lie in an exquisitely comfortable reclining chair in a quiet, dimly lit room. The therapist helps you to relax conversationally or sometimes through imagery, such as asking you to imagine sinking slowly in warm sand. The machine keeps you informed about how relaxed you are. For example, it might sound a buzzer that is high-pitched when you're tense but sinks to a lower and lower pitch as your muscles let go.

The sound is the feedback. You receive some feedback from your own muscles, but their signal is not as clear. You may not be aware that your jaw is clenched, your shoulders hunched, until the level of your tension is buzzed to you by the biofeedback machine. As you practice lowering the pitch of the buzzer, you learn to relax completely. After only a few biofeedback sessions, you can sense internal signals of your muscle tension more clearly and can from then on relax when you wish, without the machine's help.

until you've learned it well. Like any new skill, that of relaxing must be practiced until it becomes easy, smooth, rhythmical, automatic — and effective. That, of course, takes time.

Vacations All Year Long

Time is what many of us struggle with the most. Remember how long summer lasted in our childhood? Summer is a fleeting season now. Children live in the moment; we're always ahead of ourselves, drowning the moment in a wash of apprehension about the future, thinking Friday when it's only Monday, scrunching the days under the same pressure with which we scrunch our backs. I've heard that time stretches out again with retirement; I hope so. Meanwhile, what can we do to numb our sense that time is rushing, running out, leaving deadlines like corpses in its wake? Here are some time-stretching techniques that have worked for others.

More and more people are trading the traditional two-week summer vacation for a series of long weekends spread through the year. That sounds relaxing to me. You don't go as far or spend as much or work as hard at squeezing the last drop of pleasure from a single trip. A long weekend can be taken at short notice. So it rains; there'll be another weekend coming up. So it was the shore this time; it will be the mountains next. Counting national holidays, you could give yourself a nice vacation nearly every month.

Another time-stretcher has been made possible by the flourishing of personal computers. One firm I know recently replaced its old PCs with new ones. The boss offered the old ones free to employees who wanted to work at home sometimes. Half the hassle of one's working day is the constant interruption, complaint, and frenzy that passes for "atmosphere" in offices. Working at home is more relaxed and, since a task is often done more quickly without colleagues looking over your shoulder and air conditioners pouring cold air down your neck, you can sleep longer in the morning and quit earlier in the afternoon — all without battling traffic or train schedules. Several workers in that office now come in four days a week instead of five and still get their assignments in on time.

The same office — and I must say it's an admirable one — also allows flexible scheduling. Some people choose to beat the rush hour both ways by starting work at eight and quitting at four. Some take a two-hour lunch break and make up the difference before or after the usual working day. Some work longer hours every day for fewer days a week.

These are just suggestions. Maybe you're Scrooge; maybe you work for him. I'm sure old Ebenezer had a stiff neck; I know Bob Cratchit had an aching back.

After a day of buffeting amid a storm of paper, one longs to sail into the harbor of one's home. Homecoming used to be a ritual, and I think it still should be. There were hot baths, slippers, canapés, and wine. True, there were also those who served, whether wives or hirelings. Homes are self-service now. Still, the little while it takes to bathe, change, and set out a tasty treat is a small investment for an hour's perfect relaxation before dinner.

Somehow it was common knowledge in those pragmatic times that a glass of wine or spirits before the evening meal settled the day's butterflies and let conversation flow. These beneficent effects of modest quantities of alcohol have only recently been rediscovered — and in nursing homes, of all places. I can't imagine how much money is spent these days on studies to rediscover the obvious. A drink before dinner, this particular study announced, enhances sociability, improves appetite, and relieves depression among the elderly.

Among all of us, I'd say.

Next they'll be telling us to soak in a hot tub, to take off our shoes, to slip into a comfy bathrobe, to invite a friend for dinner, to take a stroll. Another study recently certified that sex remains enjoyable at any age. Who would have guessed?

At our age, we don't need psychologists to tell us that friendly people are less tense than antisocial ones, that good marriages make couples happy, that optimism is healthier than pessimism, that old age is most pleasantly spent by those who have been satisfied with their lives. Such truisms are no more helpful in a practical sense than the statement "Relax; you'll feel better."

We may, however, need to be reminded to count our blessings. There are pleasures in the second half of life that weren't available before and that are downright relaxing.

For many of us, children are grown and gone, along with their dirty socks and squabbles and our duty to raise them well. Trivia annoy us less; we waste less time hassling friends or spouses toward some standard of perfection that, by now, pales before endearingly familiar eccentricities. We have more to talk about: more than half a century of observations, experiences, knowledge, and memory. We no longer fear that the world depends solely on our energy and idealism for its salvation. We've become efficient: We cook without creating heaps of greasy dishes, write more succinctly, speak more to the point, and marshal facts more accurately than the young. Call it dignity; call it wisdom: A pimple on the chin can no longer make us nearly suicidal. We're not scrabbling so urgently up the ladder of success that someone could make us work a ninety-hour week, as up-and-coming lawyers are made to do, as young doctors do routinely, as young couples holding down four jobs between them must do if they are ever to buy the house they will at last come home to.

We're home. We can relax.

And take pleasure in the strength and vigor that will let us count our blessings in fitness and in health for many years to come.